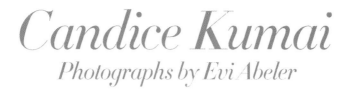

Candice Kumai
Photographs by Evi Abeler

CLEAN GREEN DRINKS

100+

Cleansing Recipes
To Renew & Restore
Your Body and Mind

GALVANIZED

NOTICE

The recommendations in this book are not meant
to diagnose or treat any medical disease or
condition. You must not rely on the information
in this book as an alternative to medical advice
from your physician or health care professional.
If you have any specific questions about any
medical matter, please consult your physician
or health care professional.

Published in the United States by
Galvanized Books, a division of
Galvanized Brands, LLC, New York

Galvanized Books is a trademark of
Galvanized Brands, LLC

DESIGN BY MIKE SMITH
PHOTOGRAPHY BY EVI ABELER

COVER PHOTOGRAPH AND
PAGES 8, 128, AND 149
BY JAMES DIMMOCK

PRINTED IN THE UNITED STATES OF AMERICA
ON ACID-FREE PAPER

ISBN 9780553390834

GALVANIZED

For Jade,

You're the perfect
shade of green
in my life. Thank
you for being my
light.
xo Chandler

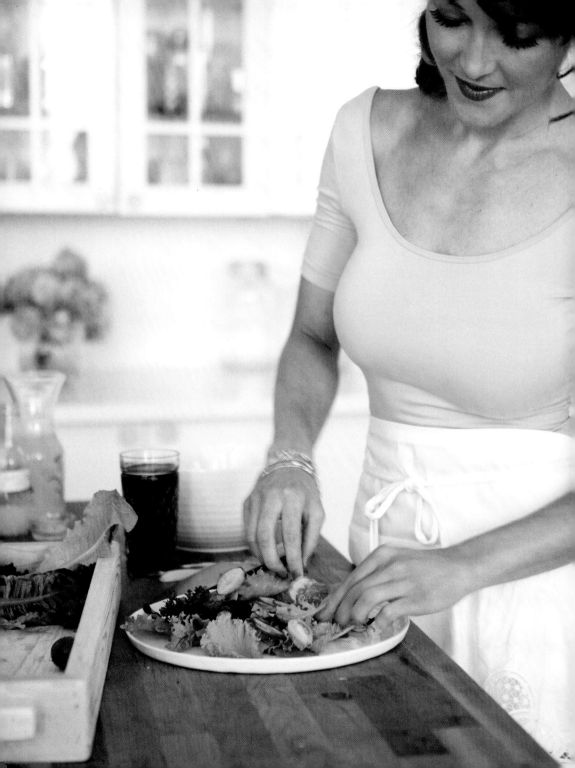

CONTENTS

Introduction:
Clean, Green, Healthy & Lean for Life! **1**

1 The Clean Green Life Guide **9**
Discover new pathways to the ultimate nutrition solution and better health.

2 Meet the Superfoods:
Getting to Know Your Ingredients **23**
Discover the natural, nutrient-dense ingredients of Clean Green drinks that
can change your life!

the recipes

3 Cleansing Juices & Smoothies **57**

4 Morning Starter Juices & Smoothies **75**

5 Filling Juices & Smoothies **91**

6 Super Energy-Boosting Juices & Smoothies **105**

7 Post-Workout Lean-Protein Smoothies **119**

8 Skin-Cleansing Juices & Smoothies **133**

9 Superfood Brain-Boosting Smoothies **151**

10 Happy, Flat Tummy Juices & Smoothies **161**

11 Body & Mind: Calming Juices & Smoothies **171**

12 Immunity-Boosting Juices & Smoothies **187**

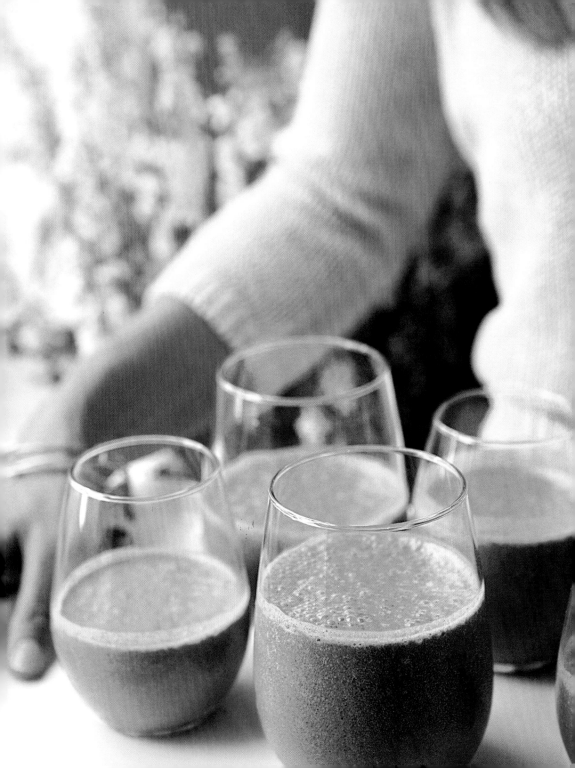

CLEAN, GREEN, HEALTHY & LEAN FOR LIFE

W ith the push of a button, your life is going to change.

You're going to transform your body, boost your health, and—odd as it may seem—improve your whole outlook on life. And it will be *easier* than you've ever imagined.

As a chef, cooking show host, cookbook author, and dedicated health journalist, I have studied the connections between nutrition, physical and emotional health, and weight loss for more than a decade. What I've learned—and what science bears out time and again—is that losing weight, looking great, and living a long, healthy life comes from two simple moves: cutting down on calories and doubling up on nutrition. Simply put, fewer calories consumed equals fewer pounds to gain. More nutrition equals less hunger. And that's a very positive thing.

Yet achieving that Holy Grail of health isn't easy. Because while you want to take in as many vitamins and minerals as possible, you also want to do it in the fewest calories possible and from whole foods. Yet, in today's society, where an estimated 70 percent of our daily calories come from heavily processed foods, that can be difficult.

That's why this book will change your life. Consider it your insider's guide to perfect nutrition; an ideal plan for maximizing nutrients, minimizing calories, and telling hunger to peace out—for good.

Why Clean Green Drinks?

GREEN IS THE NEW BLACK. The green and organic juice market has grown to a multi-billion dollar industry, and it's expected to continue booming. Companies are cashing in, with many consumers willing to cough up $10-plus for a clean-green fix. As celebrities, health gurus, and foodies the world over tout juicing as the new hot thing, sporting a green drink has become somewhat of a status symbol. But it's not just a fad. The proven nutritional benefits of sipping green are numerous and far outweigh its sex appeal.

In fact, juices for healing date back to ancient societies around the world. In the Biblical era, juicing remedies found in Dead Sea Scrolls were promoted by the Essenes. Ancient Indian writings sing the praises healing drinks made from vegetables, fruits, and herbs. The Ayurvedic term *amit ras*, roughly translates to "immortality juice" and speaks to the ability of such natural elixirs to optimize life's energy.

Research continues to prove that consuming more fresh produce is one of the easiest and most realistic ways to achieve and maintain a healthy weight, not to mention overall well-being! And the easiest way to ensure you're getting your fill of nutrition-packed produce is to whip up a selection of gorgeous greens into a delicious drink that takes, literally, seconds to sip. (Although, these recipes are so terrific, you'll want to savor them!)

Just take a look at what science tells us about the benefits of the juices and smoothies like those you'll enjoy in this book:

1 You'll get top nutrition. Vegetables and fruits contribute vital

vitamins and antioxidants to your body, and the vast majority of us aren't getting enough. A 2013 study by the Centers for Disease Control and Prevention found that adults in the United States consume fruit about 1.1 times per day and vegetables about 1.6 times per day—far below the recommended daily servings of at least four and three, respectively. Juicing is the easiest way to get a high volume of fruits and veggies into your bod, and a variety at that! Consider this: We would need to eat two pounds of carrots, 10 to 12 apples, or eight pounds of spinach to get the same amount of nutrients found in 16 ounces of produce-packed juice. Amazing!

2 You can lose and manage weight naturally.

Juicing isn't just about weight loss, but better-fitting jeans can be a happy side effect. That's because most fruits and vegetables are low in energy density due to their high water and fiber content, and low fat content. Researchers at Baylor College of Medicine found that dieters who drank an eight-ounce glass of low-sodium vegetable juice daily over a 12-week period lost, on average, four pounds more than dieters who did not drink the juice.

3 Your digestive system will thank you. Since juicing strips produce of its fiber, your body gets a leg up on digestion. And unlike many bottled drinks that are heated during pasteurization and sometimes hide both synthetic and genetically modified ingredients, fresh juices are totally raw and you control what goes in them. It's believed that consuming raw produce boosts digestion by preserving vital enzymes, which means less bloat and more regular bowel movements, for a flat, happy belly!

4 You'll feel calmer and happier. Studies suggest that eating more fresh produce has a positive effect on mood. Researchers from University of Otago's department of human nutrition evaluated the relationship between day-to-day emotions and food consumption and found that participants felt happier, calmer, and more positive on days when they consumed fruits and vegetables.

5 You'll think more clearly. Studies show that raw foods, especially vitamin- and antioxidant-rich fruit and vegetable juices, can boost brain function by reducing the damage caused to brain cells. A 2006 Vanderbilt University study found that people who consumed three or more servings of fruit and vegetable juice each week were 76 percent less likely to develop signs of Alzheimer's over 10 years than those who drank fewer than one serving a week. Clean, green, and keen!

6 You'll have better sex. Diet affects our libido in numerous ways, and you can, quite literally, juice up your sex life. Some foods, like chili peppers, ginger, garlic, and avocados, actually increase blood flow to the genitals. Wowza! There are fertility benefits of a diet high in fruits and vegetables, as well. Researchers at Harvard University pointed out that extra iron from plants such as spinach improve a woman's baby-making prospects. And research from the University of Texas Medical Branch found that men who consume at least 200 milligrams of vitamin C a day can improve their sperm counts and motility. Who needs pills when you can juice?!

7 **You'll have more energy.** Your body's vitality and endurance are closely related to a proper pH balance. The body's entire metabolic process depends on an alkaline environment, which is often interrupted by the typical highly acidic American diet. Fresh fruits and vegetables can counter the effects due to their high alkalinity. A healthy pH balance means more pep in your step!

8 **You'll glow.** Hey, gorgeous, would you believe that you can get the same benefits from juicing as you might from a top-dollar facial? I've dedicated an entire chapter of this book to skin-saving drinks (page 132), brimming with vitamins and minerals proven to improve your skin's health. And check this out: A recent study in Scotland suggests carotenoids, the highly pigmented compounds found in most produce, can actually increase the yellow and red tones in your skin, resulting in a more even glow. (Beauty starts on the inside. Pass it on.)

9 **You'll sleep better.** Adequate, high-quality sleep is essential for mental health, hormonal balance, and recovery. According to the National Sleep Foundation, more than half of American adults experience a sleep problem a few nights a week, and the culprit is often a deficiency in essential nutrients. Juicing can help you meet daily requirements for sleep-enhancing vitamins and minerals.

10 **You'll have fun!** Anything I can juice, you can juice better. Really. You don't need a culinary background to create a gorgeously green juice or smoothie. And you don't need a bushel of exotic produce to start, either. The recipes in this book are easy and accessible; many can be made with ingredients you may already have in your fridge. You'll enjoy the creative process of experimenting with different recipes and flavor combinations. It's instantly rewarding. Plus, what's more fun than looking and feeling better?

And the story begins...

Get all of these benefits simply by enjoying one or two of these delicious Clean Green drinks daily. That's it. So rather than feeling burdened to eat your veggies, now you can drink them instead! No rules. Just start juicing and blending, and see how you feel.

Maybe you've tried a few juices before and found the taste somewhat...lacking. I totally understand, and believe me, I'm as much a hedonist as anyone. I wouldn't subject my taste buds to anything that wasn't delicious, and I won't do that to yours, either. After all, as a judge on *Iron Chef America*, my job is to get tough on chefs who don't tickle my taste buds (which is rare!). However, the cook I'm toughest on is myself.

Still, I'm innately dedicated to fresh, healthy eating. I was raised by a wonderful Japanese mother who was born into a life of eating produce straight from the organic soil, in southern Japan. There, while she was teaching, she met my American father, who was serving in the U.S. Navy at the time. Despite their cultural and religious differences, love still conquered all, and she later moved to the U.S. in the 1970s to marry him.

For more than thirty years now, she has been a devoted Japanese language teacher, wife, and mom. She shares her beloved heritage and Clean Green lifestyle with all of her students and my sister and me. ("Yes, Kumai Sensei!") My father is a hardworking, philanthropic man who was born and raised on a farm in Poland. He immigrated to the U.S. when he was just eleven years old, to later earn a degree from Hartford Tech and serve in the U.S. Navy. He became an engineer and, eventually, an energy-conserving activist and professional auditor with Southern California Edison for decades.

I grew up alongside my smart-as-a-whip, Berkeley grad, tatted-up older sister, Jenni, who has dedicated the past 20 years of her life to "green" philanthropy. Now the director and founder of her own nonprofit go-green cycling shop, the London Bike Kitchen, Jenni's award-winning bike shop was named by the London Cycling

Awards for best community project within its first year of opening. (Brava, sis!)

My family's calling and life's goal is to do good and share the love of the "go-green" lifestyle in every way we can. I have traveled and explored family farms across the U.S.—in Hawaii; Napa Valley; Ohio; Miami; New York; Washington, D.C.; Dallas; San Diego; and Los Angeles—learning about the soil that forms America's roots. I find it absolutely invigorating to meet others who are sharing their stories and growing this beautiful nation together. And while the past decade of my life includes television (from *Top Chef* to *Cook Yourself Thin* to *Iron Chef America*), digital media, and publishing, they are just the "green" icing on my cake; they're not at the heart of my work. The heart of my work is in helping people improve their lives!

And that's why I want you to go clean and green.

I was once told by a doctor that we'll all be in our own rocking chair one day, asking ourselves, "Did I have a great time? Did I love my life?" You'll want to say, "Hell yeah, and I lived clean, green, and lean!" This book is your investment for the long term.

Confidence is the key to success in any field, including your nutrition. If you think you can, you absolutely will. Make a positive commitment to focus on change and reveal your abs, boost your energy, and claim the life you want!

Remember, beauty always starts from the inside. Reveal your true self. Be clean; be green.

XX Candice

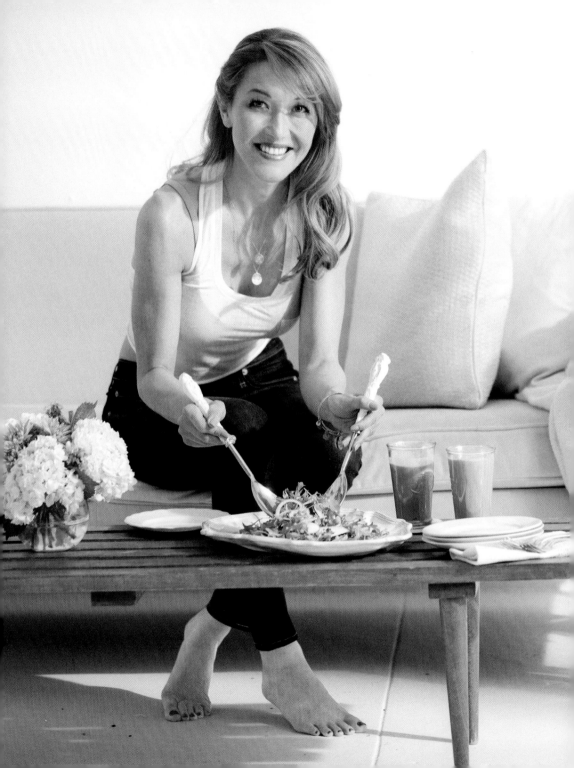

The Clean Green Life Guide

THIS BOOK IS about two things: proper nutrition and satiety. They work hand-in-hand to keep you lean, healthy, and happy. If there's one thing I want you to take away from this book, it's the definition of these two words:

Nutrition: nu·tri·tion

noun \nu̇-'tri-shən, nyu̇-\ : the process of eating the right kind of food so you can grow properly and be healthy. (SOURCE: MERRIAM-WEBSTER)

Satiety: sa·ti·ety

noun \sə -'tī- ə-tē *also* 'sā-sh(ē-) ə-\ : a feeling or condition of being full after eating food. (SOURCE: MERRIAM-WEBSTER)

My ultimate goal is to inspire you to seek out proper nutrition through real foods while simultaneously learning to master and embrace the feelings of hunger and satiety—and to tell the difference between them. The first step toward being happy and satisfied is to teach yourself what it's like to experience these feelings. You'll learn how in *Clean Green Drinks*.

First, let me answer a few questions and walk you through some of the terms that might come up in this book.

QUESTION #1

What's the difference between juices and smoothies?

Juices contain fruits and vegetables only. A proper juicing machine (see page 50) extracts the juice from whole produce and removes the pulp, leaving just its vitamins and minerals. Freshly made juices are bursting with nutrients that naturally strengthen your immune system and help prevent disease. The Clean Green juices you'll make using this book are just that. But make sure to limit the amount of fruit added (watch out for those sugars!), a frequent pitfall that *Clean Green Drinks* side-steps completely.

Juices are also easier to digest than smoothies because the pulp and roughage are removed, and are thus helpful for those with sensitive digestive systems. Juicing should be used to nourish, cleanse, and rejuvenate the body.

Smoothies contain fruits and vegetables and their roughage, plus ice, liquids (page 46), protein powders, and/or supplements or super-boosters (page 40). These ingredients are placed into a high-powered blender (see page 53 for the best equipment) and blended until smooth. (Hence, the word "smoothie.") Blended smoothies retain their fiber and contain extra vitamins, minerals, and phytochemicals derived from the skin, peel, and pith of the produce. Drinking smoothies can help you learn about the feeling of proper satiety, thanks to their fiber.

But be careful: Your typical supermarket or food-chain "smoothie" may be more of a "milkshake" than a nutritious meal. Some smoothie chains and fast-food joints add excess sugar, calories, frozen yogurt, ice cream, and other extras that aren't waist-friendly! That's exactly why I want to show you how easy it is to make your own.

The Clean Green smoothies you'll find in this book will kick-start your health and get you back to a clean base of nutrition to help you reach and maintain a healthy weight.

—————

Isn't this expensive? I can't afford to juice and make smoothies. I'm on a budget.

Too often juicing gets a bad rap for being an elitist diet that will leave you pinching pennies. Living the Clean Green lifestyle is an investment, for sure, but it may not be the wallet squeeze you're anticipating. In fact, juicing Clean Green drinks on the regular can actually save you money. I've crunched the numbers, and the cost per serving for most recipes in this book is under $4. That's a savings of up to $6 on the most popular bottled juices; even more if you're signing up for a cleanse.

The markup on commercially produced juices and smoothies is significant. Not only are juice companies funding the cost of production, but many menus and products rely on the year-round availability of specific ingredients, which runs up food costs and retail price. Berries, for example, can be wildly expensive out of season.

Let's not forget that while the price of a bottled beverage spikes, the nutritional value can take a dip. Pasteurization processes that preserve a drink's freshness can affect its enzymatic properties in unpredictable ways. And some bottled drinks contain additives that compromise their cleanness and greenness.

Not a bottled-smoothie buyer, you say? Well consider the average working lunch. A recent survey from Visa shows Americans eat out for lunch twice per week on average and spend just under $10 each outing, averaging about $18 a week, and adding up to $936 a year. For that money you could be sipping on multiple green juices each week, and fund the cost of a high-end juicer.

But the real value lies in the health benefits. Clean Green juices and smoothies actually pay you back. You're investing in a leaner, calmer, happier, and more energized you. The average cost of one of my Clean Green drinks? $4. The cost of your health? Priceless.

How can I commit to Clean Green smoothies and juices at the office or while traveling?

If you truly commit to this change, you can realistically commit to this lifestyle 75–80 percent of the time. I have friends who take their Magic Bullet Blender or NutriBullet to work (see equipment on page 50); or, their office chipped in to purchase a juicer or blender to have in the break room. Another great option: Purchase a BlenderBottle, fill it with a fresh smoothie or juice you made at home, and consume within two hours of blending or juicing. I usually blend one and sip it on my way to work or yoga.

While traveling through Japan for a few weeks, I brought along my NutriBullet and used it in my hotel and at my grandma's place. It wasn't a pain; it was actually just an extra item in my suitcase. While traveling, you too can certainly stick to this regimen. To make it easier, purchase a small, handheld immersion blender. All you'll need to pack are your superfood greens, spirulina, and protein powders in resealable bags; the rest is fresh. And don't forget to pack this book with you; it's one of the reasons

WHEN TO BUY
ORGANIC

DIRTY DOZEN

According to the Environmental Working Group's 2013 Shopper's Guide to Pesticides in Produce, the following popular fresh produce was analyzed and found to carry the most pesticide residue. (*Testing data from the U.S. Department of Agriculture and the Food and Drug Administration.*) The dozen listed here are ranked from worst to best (lower numbers = more pesticides).

1. Apples
2. Strawberries
3. Grapes
4. Celery
5. Peaches
6. Spinach
7. Sweet Bell Peppers
8. Nectarines (imported)
9. Cucumbers
10. Potatoes
11. Cherry Tomatoes
12. Hot Peppers

CLEAN FIFTEEN

According to the EWG's Clean Fifteen list for 2013, the following popular fresh produce items are least likely to test positive for pesticide residues so are safe to purchase non-organic, due to their husks, peels, and skins. (*Testing data from USDA and FDA.*)

1. Asparagus
2. Avocados
3. Cabbage
4. Cantaloupe
5. Sweet Corn
6. Eggplant
7. Grapefruits
8. Kiwis
9. Mangoes
10. Mushrooms
11. Onions
12. Papayas
13. Pineapples
14. Sweet Peas (frozen)
15. Sweet Potatoes

I made it handbook size!

Or, heck, you can simply enjoy your vacation for a week or two and live it up! These Clean Green drinks are so effective at reversing the sins of your diet that you can fully embrace holidays, birthdays, and vacations and then get back on track with a few days of juicing.

Why the emphasis on consuming Clean Green drinks immediately?

When it comes to juicing, time is of the essence. In fact, Clean Green drinks are best consumed within 20 minutes of juicing. Here's why: From the moment juices are exposed to air, their enzymatic and nutritional value begin to deteriorate. It's a process known as oxidation, which is simply exposure to oxygen. Think about a freshly cut apple that browns over time or a ripening banana. Blended juices and smoothies are even more susceptible to oxidation, since every part of the produce has been exposed to air. Because of this, store-bought bottled juices are pasteurized to prevent oxidation and preserve freshness. Not only will the nutritional value of your juice diminish over time, but the taste might also take a hit. (You've been warned...)

CENTRIFUGAL VS. MASTICATING:

Centrifugal juicers use a spinning blade, which creates heat that can destroy precious nutrients and enzymes. My best advice when using centrifugal juicers is to juice and drink immediately, so you don't sell yourself short on nutrients.

Masticating juicers use a "chewing" or "crushing" type of force to press juice, with zero heat. Thus you will receive the most nutrient content from juices pressed with a masticating juicer. Hurom, Omega, and Norwalk are three brands to check out, or see page 50.

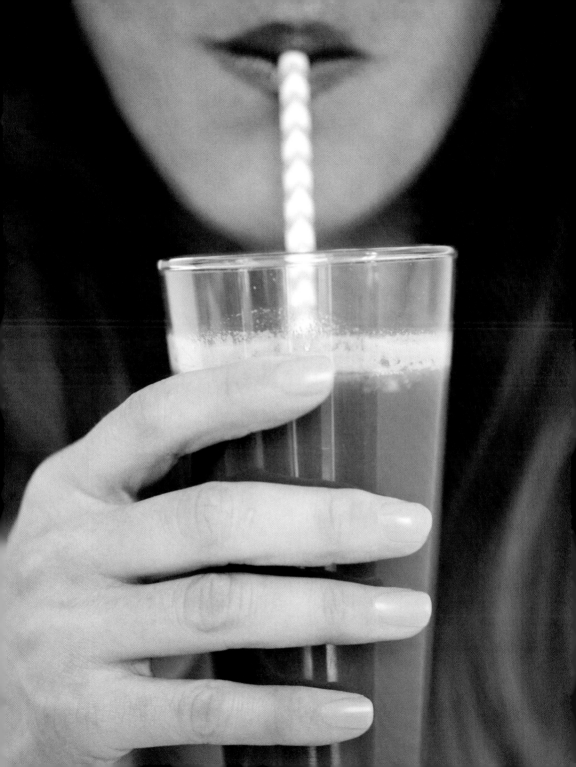

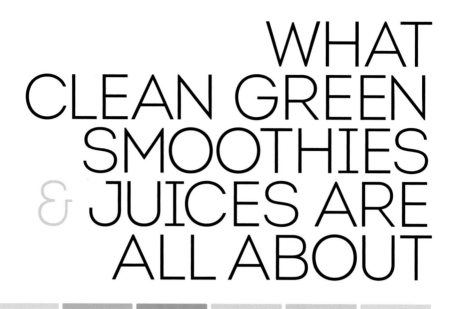

WHAT CLEAN GREEN SMOOTHIES & JUICES ARE ALL ABOUT

Low in Sugar

These drinks have fewer calories and sugars than most store-bought drinks. My Açaí Super Berry (page 115) has 130 calories and 10 grams of natural sugar, whereas the equivalent at a popular smoothie chain could cost you twice the calories and upwards of 40 grams of sugar! Less sugar also means fewer blood-sugar spikes, which are ultimately responsible for those midday "crashes" among other things.

Unprocessed

Clean Green drinks are all natural and contain fewer ingredients, no chemicals, no additives, and no preservatives. I am all about going back to the Clean Green basics.

Protein-Packed

Protein is the source of your lean, toned muscles that burn fat while keeping you strong. It's also digested more slowly than the other macronutrients (i.e., fats and carbs), so it will keep you feeling fuller longer. Most of the smoothies you'll find in the Post-Workout Lean Protein Smoothies chapter (page 118) were designed for you to consume after exercising, when you need protein most.

Fiber-Filled

Fiber helps aid digestion, keeps you regular, and keeps you fuller longer. My smoothies pack a roughage punch, since they retain all the pulp and fibrous cellulose that's removed by a juicer. Add in chia seeds, flaxseeds, spirulina, and other natural green superfoods for an extra filling, naturally cleansing boost!

Nutrient-Dense

These Clean Green juices and smoothies are packed with vitamins, minerals, and anti-oxidants—not calories, fat, or sugar. It's not easy to snack on kale, spinach, or spirulina at the office, on the road, or during a parent-teacher conference; but you can quickly blend superfoods into a smoothie or juice and get your fill of Clean Green goodness.

Gluten-Free

My receipes are wheat-free, gluten-free, and easy for all bodies to digest. Between 5 and 10 percent of all people may suffer from a gluten sensitivity of some form, and some studies have shown that cutting wheat and gluten may be beneficial to a slim physique. Gluten can also spike blood sugar levels, and may lead to inflammation; so I simply choose to stay away from it. Let's start this journey gluten-free.

Low in Dairy

Occasionally, you'll see my love for Greek yogurt prevail, and I use whey protein, too, which is a byproduct of cheese. However, you will not see dairy milk in this book. Around 12 percent of the population considers itself lactose intolerant, whether medically confirmed or self-diagnosed. Dairy can be hard on the tummy; almond milk and coconut milk are great alternatives. Unsweetened almond and coconut milk are also low in sugar, and at only 35 to 45 calories a cup? You can't beat that.

CLEAN GREEN EATING & EXERCISE GUIDE

Exercise Clean Green

Exercise is an essential part of the Clean Green life. In all of my research—from personal to case studies to new books, diets, and magazines—working out seems to be the key to a longer, healthier, and happier life.

In fact, a recently published study in *British Medical Journal* showed exercise to be just as effective as drugs in treating those with heart disease and those at high risk of diabetes. And physical activity was even more effective than medication for certain groups; researchers suggest prescribing exercise instead of drugs to stroke patients could revolutionize their health.

And for mental health, too, exercise can be hugely rewarding. Having a bad day? In a study at the University of Texas that explored exercise as a treatment for serious depression, participants mentioned that they felt happier after a brisk 30-minute sweat sesh. Break a sweat and beat the blues, my friend!

My favorite ways to workout are in the following chart: yoga, running, and the Bar Method. Along with mind-clearing meditation, find a workout that works for your beautiful bod and reap all of the benefits!

Clean Green Eating

Here's a week's worth of menus for you to try! For breakfast and lunch, mix and match Clean Green juices and smoothies throughout the week, and cook up a clean meal for dinner. Also drink 8–10 glasses of water daily. For more recipes, check out *candicekumai.com*.

	MONDAY	TUESDAY	WEDNESDAY
BREAKFAST	The Chocolate Morning Wake-up Smoothie p.82	The Breakfast Blend Smoothie p.88	The Green Matcha Tea Smoothie p.86
LUNCH	The Blueberry Super-Immunity Booster Smoothie p.194	The Super Hemp Smoothie p.131	The Honeydew Mint Refresher Smoothie p.182
ENERGY-BOOSTING JUICE	The Sour Apple Juice p.65	The Kale Apple Juice p.92	The Super Charger Juice p.194
AFTERNOON SNACK & EVENING WORKOUT/ MEDITATION	1 apple with 1 tbsp cashew butter & Yoga	¼ cup roasted cashews & (Workout) Bar Method	½ avocado with soy sauce and lemon & Meditation/Running
DINNER For recipes, visit candicekumai.com	Quinoa & Clean Greens Salad	Roasted Corn and Heirloom Tomato Salad	Brussels Sprout Clean Green Salad
BEDTIME	Herbal tea: Yogi Calming tea	Homemade herbal tea: fresh rosemary with a touch of honey	Homemade herbal tea: mint-chamomile

& Exercise Guide

And yes, you CAN snack mindfully! Here are a few of my favorite Clean Green treats to hold you over in your first few weeks: ¼ cup cashews or almonds, ½ avocado with soy sauce and lemon, 1 banana, 1 apple with almond butter, or organic fruit and nut bars.

THURSDAY	FRIDAY	SATURDAY	SUNDAY
The Green Sunshine Smoothie p.88	The Green Banana-Mint Smoothie p.95	The Cinnamon Almond Horchata Smoothie p.113	The Chocolate Avocado Goddess Smoothie p.178
The Creamy Pumpkin Pie Smoothie p.142	The Blueberry Protein Power "Shake" p.120	The Clean Green Tea Smoothie p.159	The Chocolate Peanut Butter Monster Smoothie p.126
The Cucumber-Mint-Coconut Cleanser Juice p.136	The Green Cucumber Cleanser Juice p.162	The Spicy-Ginger Pineapple Green Juice p.110	The Lavender-Melon Refresher Juice p.173
1 apple with 1 tbsp almond butter & (Workout) Bar Method	Organic fruit and nut bars (e.g., Kind Bar) & Meditation	1 banana with 1 tbsp almond butter & (Workout) Bar Method	2 Nibmor dark chocolate squares, ½ cup pumpkin seeds & Meditation/ Running
Clean Green Flatbread Pizza!	Candice's Cleansing Carrot Ginger Soup or Cleansing Cold Cucumber Soup	Clean Green Roasted Spaghetti Squash	Clean Green Eggs over Gluten-Free Toast
Herbal tea: lavender with a touch of honey	Herbal tea: Yogi Peach Detox tea	Herbal tea: Celestial Seasonings Sleepytime tea	Homemade herbal tea: pineapple, ginger, and honey

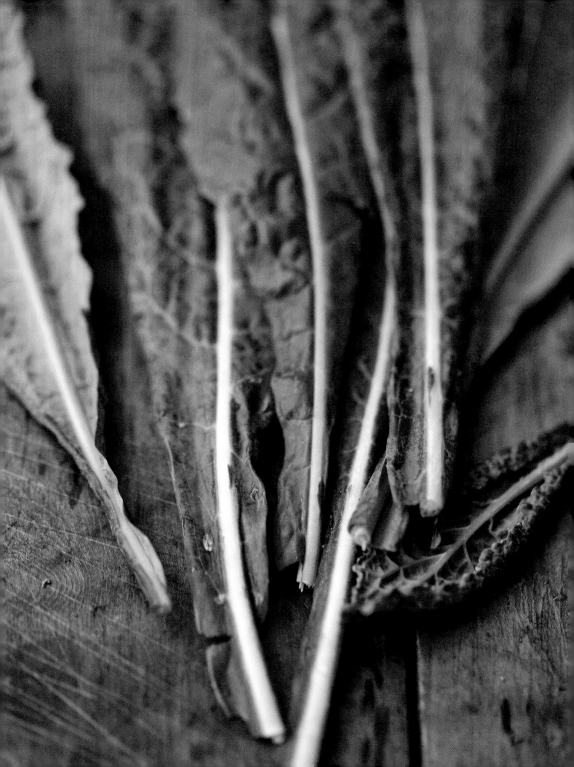

Meet the Superfoods: Getting to Know Your Ingredients

2

ONE OF THE great things about juicing is that you know exactly what you're putting into your body—something most of us simply can't claim on a daily basis. Nowadays, something as simple as bread can have, literally, dozens of ingredients; and basic restaurant fare like a single hamburger can clock in at a full day's recommended intake of calories. Yuck.

But in this chapter, you're going to discover the simple, from-the-earth ingredients that make up Clean Green drinks, and learn how they can help change your life, your health, and your outlook on a cleaner, greener future.

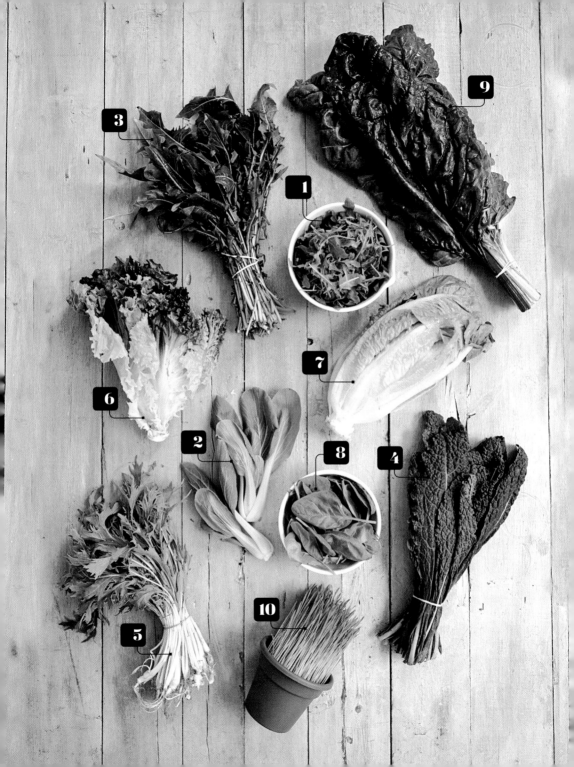

MEET THE GREENS!

The sassiest, greenest leaves also happen to be the most nutrient-dense. Get your green on! It looks so vibrant on you! Note: Organic is truly best, so purchase it whenever possible.

(Check out the "Dirty Dozen" and "Clean Fifteen" on page 13 for guidelines.)

THE GREENS

1 Arugula
2 Bok Choy
3 Dandelion Greens
4 Kale
5 Mizuna
6 Red Leaf Lettuce
7 Romaine
8 Spinach
9 Swiss Chard
10 Wheat Grass

1 Arugula (aka Rocket)

My favorite salad and flatbread topping, arugula is also simple to juice and blend. Containing iron; calcium; fiber; protein; vitamins A, C, E, and K; as well as phytochemicals such as beta-carotene, this supergreen can be used in place of spinach in any of these Clean Green drinks.

2 Bok Choy

With a substantial amount of calcium; potassium; and vitamins A, B6, C, and E, this favorite in Asia is high in water content, which makes it ideal for juicing. Don't limit it to stir-fries anymore.

3 Dandelion Greens

Need more iron, calcium, fiber, protein, and vitamins A, B6, C, E, and K? Try dandelion greens! These bitter greens are certainly an acquired taste, so be sure to test them out prior to serving at your next brunch. Despite their bitterness, they are packed with nutrients and work well when juiced with sweet fruits or blended with bananas.

4 Kale

A super-mega-green, kale might be the most-talked-about green on the market. Loaded with cancer-fighting nutrients like iron; calcium; protein; potassium; vitamins A, B6, and C; carotenoids; lutein; and phytochemicals, it's no wonder this once-overlooked green has become the star of the show! I love blending lacinato kale (or dinosaur kale) into my smoothies and juicing with this supergreen in the A.M. You just radiate from an inner "kale glow."

5 Mizuna

Full of iron, calcium, fiber, protein, and vitamins A, B6, and C, this Japanese mustard green is one of my favorites to wake up a boring old salad. Try mizuna whipped up in a smoothie, or juice away with this clean, mean green.

6 Red Leaf Lettuce

My mom's favorite green contains calcium, protein, and vitamins A, B6, C, and E. This lettuce is a favorite of mine to add to fresh juices. And its water content makes it perfect.

7 Romaine

Not just for Caesar salads anymore, romaine boasts iron, calcium, potassium, and vitamins A, B6, and C. Romaine is also packed with fiber to make for a happy tummy.

8 Spinach

This supergreen is the most utilized ingredient in *Clean Green Drinks*. It has a great low price and "neatness"; spinach is also easy to measure, with no chopping needed (1 handful of baby spinach or arugula = approximately 1 cup. See page 103 for more greens measuring tips). Bonus for kids: You can barely taste it! Spinach is also packed with iron; calcium; protein; vitamins A, B6, C, E; fiber; and phytochemicals like beta-carotene, lutein, and folate. When this green is combined with citrus like lemon or orange, you can boost its nutritional absorption.

9 Swiss Chard

Packed with iron, calcium, fiber, and vitamins A, B6, C, E, and K, Swiss chard is easy to juice and blend. A study by the Institute of Food Technology in Germany found Swiss chard to be loaded with glutamine, an amino acid that boosts the immune system and aids the healing of wounds.

11 Wheat Grass

Full of antioxidants, vitamins, minerals, enzymes, and chlorophyll, wheat grass is a total superfood that can be found at your local health food store and at most farmer's markets. Just trim with a pair of clean kitchen shears, and juice with apple or pear and a little cucumber. You can even share a little with your pets (*mee-ow!*).

TIPS FOR STORING YOUR GREENS

Immediately pick through your greens and rid the bunch of any bad leaves.

Keep your greens as dry as possible after rinsing. You can wrap greens in a dry paper towel and keep them in a plastic bag or container in the fridge. Alternatively—and here's a tip I borrowed from Jamie Oliver—turn your bottom fridge drawer into a greens basket by lining it with a clean dish towel.

To revive wilted greens, try shocking them in ice water. A quick dip should perk them up right away. Drain the leaves on paper towels, or give them a quick whirl through a salad spinner.

Store your fruits and veggies separately, as many fruits contain ethylene, which causes fruits to ripen and greens to wilt.

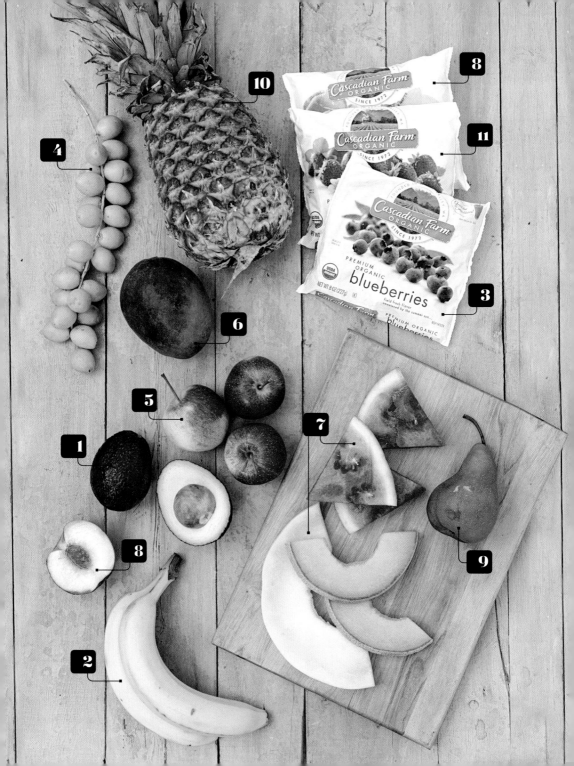

> *"Respect thy avocado. Next to chocolate, it's the best thing that Mother Nature gave us."* —CANDICE KUMAI

SUPERFRUITS

The most recommended fruits to blend and juice, to bring out the gorgeous green goddess that you are!

SUPERFRUITS

1. Avocados
2. Bananas
3. Blueberries
4. Dates
5. Apples
6. Mangoes
7. Melons
8. Peaches
9. Pears
10. Pineapple
11. Strawberries
12. Citrus Fruits (not pictured)

1 Avocados

I could not live without this decadent fruit. It is the love of my life and is quite possibly one of the best fruits to blend due to its good monounsaturated fats; plus you get a whole lot of vitamins A, C, and E, too. Avocados are synonymous with beautiful hair, skin, and nails.

2 Bananas (Fresh or Frozen)

The most commonly used fruit in my smoothie recipes, bananas, especially frozen ones, blend to a perfect consistency with other produce, making them ideal superfruits. I like to say that frozen bananas are much like nature's ice cream, without all of the bloat and guilt. You're going to get your share of potassium, folate, and vitamins B1, B3, B6, and C. Bananas also help

29

aid digestion by boosting the levels of good bacteria already present in the belly. They also help restore electrolytes, naturally! See page 39 for tips on freezing them.

3 Blueberries (Organic, Frozen)

Loaded with healthy antioxidants, these super-berries may help prevent wrinkles! Researchers at the University of Maine also found that a diet rich in wild blueberries may improve conditions associated with metabolic syndrome, including cardiovascular disease and diabetes. I love blending these gorgeous blues in the morning and post-workout. Blueberries blend beautifully with spinach and kale, and boosters like superfood greens and spirulina.

4 Dates (Fresh or Dried)

Toss two or three of these little babies into your smoothies for a touch of sweetness without any processed chemicals. Just make sure they are pitted!

5 Apples (Organic)

Fuji apples are my favorite: They're not too sweet or too tart. I love juicing with these deliciously crisp and fiber-filled treats. Or opt for varieties like Granny Smith and Gala. Apples are filled with dietary fiber, vitamin C, and antioxidants.

6 Mangoes (Organic, Fresh or Frozen)

Mango has a beautiful, creamy consistency that greatly enhances smoothies, which makes this exotic fruit one of my favorites in Clean Green drinks. Just be sure to peel before blending, and remove that big-ol' pit inside.

7 Melons

These juicy fruits add great consistency to smoothies and liquid volume to juices. I recommend everything from watermelon to honeydew to cantaloupe, just make sure not to add too much; some melons (like honeydew) contain loads of sugar.

8 **Peaches** (Organic, Fresh or Frozen)

Peaches contain key nutrients like vitamin C, fiber, magnesium, phosphorus, and beta-carotene, which can boost your immunity and eye health. Note: Frozen peaches can be tough to blend, so be sure to soften them slightly by defrosting for 15 minutes prior to blending.

9 **Pears**

Known for their ability to reduce inflammation and lower blood pressure, pears are also filled with insoluble fiber, folate, potassium, and vitamins B and C. They are naturally low in calories and make for a great base to any smoothie or juice. Pears are mild in flavor, light in color, and have a great texture.

10 **Pineapple**

Packed with enzymes like bromelain, freshly sliced pineapple is one of my favorite ways to perk up a juice or smoothie with a little punch of acidity and sweetness.

11 **Strawberries** (Organic, Fresh or Frozen)

Bursting with flavor, antioxidants, and vitamin C, strawberries add a sweet and tart flavor to your smoothies. They pair perfectly with mangoes, bananas, blueberries, or raspberries. Try them with a touch of fresh basil or mint. Remember go organic when purchasing these little gems.

12 **Citrus Fruits** (Lemons, Limes, Oranges)

Juicy, delicious, and bursting with vitamin C, citrus fruits aid the synthesis of collagen, which keeps skin beautifully elastic and helps wounds heal. Citrus fruits are also rich in flavonoids, compounds that have been shown to inhibit the growth of cancer cells and prevent the spread of tumors. The citric acid in lemons and limes acts as a natural preservative and can slow oxidation when added to your Clean Green drinks.

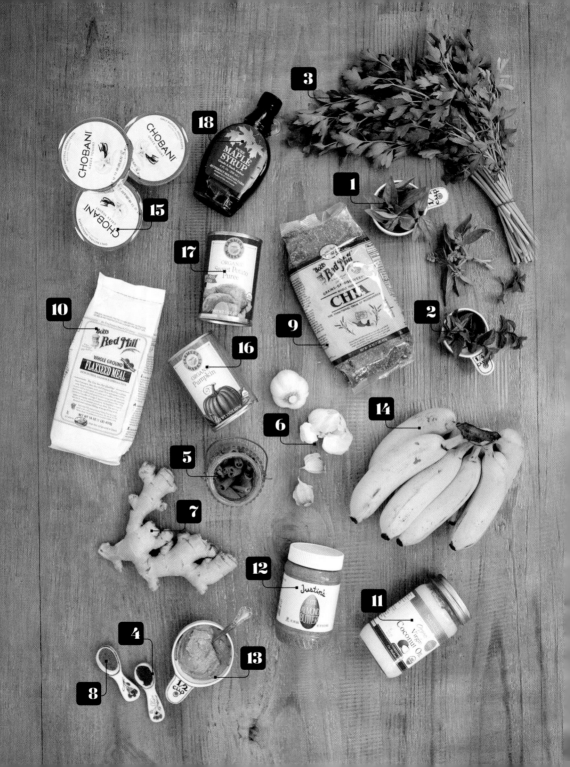

> *"To reduce inflammation in thy body. To restore thy mind. To nurture back to health."* –CK

PANTRY (& FRIDGE) RAID!

Everyday pantry staples can be used to boost your juices and smoothies for BIG results.

THE PANTRY

1. Basil
2. Mint
3. Parsley
4. Cayenne Pepper
5. Cinnamon
6. Garlic
7. Ginger
8. Nutmeg
9. Chia Seeds
10. Flaxseed & Flaxseed Meal
11. Coconut Oil
12. Natural Almond Butter
13. Natural Peanut Butter
14. Bananas
15. Greek Yogurt & Coconut Yogurt
16. Pumpkin Puree
17. Sweet Potato Puree
18. Maple Syrup

HAPPY HERBS

1 Basil

Try some of my amazing "spa-like" green drinks with the addition of fresh basil, and get a healthy dose of vitamins A and K, iron, and flavonoids. It's also great for cardiovascular health, boasts antibiotic and anti-inflammatory properties, aids in digestion, and may help ease tummyaches.

STORING JUICING HERBS

Fresh herbs can be stored like flowers at room temperature. (They're equally pretty and smell divine.) Trim the stems and place in a small vase or jar with an inch of water, just as you would a floral bouquet. To keep herbs fresh for up to a few days, cover the vase loosely with a plastic bag and store in the fridge.

STORING SPICES

Cook with the freshest spices for optimal health benefits. Most ground spices will hold for a year. After that, they lose their flavor and healing properties. Don't underestimate the power of the sniff test! If your spices are no longer fragrant, it's time to toss 'em.

2 Mint

Juicing with mint or adding it to a fresh Clean Green smoothie ain't bad, either! Packed with vitamins A and C, mint soothes upset tummies and helps aid in the treatment of irritable bowel syndrome.

3 Parsley

Parsley juices and blends well, adds major phytonutrients, and freshens breath! It's also full of vitamins A, C, and K, as well as folate, iron, and major antioxidants.

SPICES & AROMATICS

4 Cayenne Pepper

A blazing-hot flavor thanks to capsaicin, cayenne may help prevent heart attacks, ulcers, psoriasis, and pain due to arthritis. It has vitamins A, B6, C, and E; iron; folate; calcium; zinc; and fiber. Who knew cayenne was such superfood hotness?

5 Cinnamon

A lovely, fragrant spice, cinnamon is naturally filled with manganese, fiber, iron, and calcium. It may help boost memory and improve colon health; and it contains antiseptic properties, aids in digestion, and benefits the heart and kidneys.

6 Garlic

Because of its potency, garlic should be used sparingly in Clean Green drinks; although it does have major bennies, including manganese and vitamins B6 and C! Garlic also boasts antioxidant and antibacterial properties, regulates blood sugar, and keeps bones healthy.

7 Ginger

One of my favorite spices to juice up, ginger is full of antioxidants, aids in digestion, and has anti-inflammatory properties. It helps alleviate morning sickness and may relieve motion sickness, too. Ginger is a definite superfood champ in my book!

8 Nutmeg

Nutmeg is a natural anti-inflammatory that helps relieve nausea, vomiting, flatulence, and diarrhea (oh-my!). It's packed with vitamins A, B6, C, and E; calcium; iron; magnesium; folate; and fiber. I love adding just a touch to my smoothies to benefit from its many medicinal properties.

NUTS & SEEDS

9 Chia Seeds

An ancient superfood that the Aztecs prized more highly than gold, chia seeds are a great source of fiber, protein, phosphorus, manganese, antioxidants, and omega-3 fatty acids. Just two tablespoons provide five times the omega-3 content of a quarter cup of walnuts!

10 Flaxseed and Flaxseed Meal

Full of fiber, omega-3s, and monounsaturated fats, flax helps with brain function and beautiful hair, skin, and nails. It's also been proven to lower cholesterol and can help relieve hot flashes during menopause.

HEALTHY FATS

11 Coconut Oil

Chock-full of good fats and medium-chain fatty acids (MCFAs) that are easier for your body to digest than other types of fats, coconut oil is cholesterol-free, helps with thyroid and blood sugar control, and is a good moisturizer for skin and hair. I love using it to remove my makeup and to help soften my skin before bedtime.

12 Natural Almond Butter

Freshly ground organic almond butter is full of manganese and protein. Justin's produces some delicious nut butters that I love and have used for years.

13 Natural Peanut Butter

Freshly ground organic peanut butter is filled with protein, good fats, fiber, calcium, iron, folate, vitamins, and resveratrol. However, due to peanut butter's fat content, use sparingly.

14 Bananas

This smoothie star (yes, again!) is full of potassium, folate, and vitamins B1, B3, B6, and C. Bananas help maintain alkaline balance and a flat tummy. Go bananas!

15 Greek Yogurt and Coconut Yogurt

Greek yogurt has plenty of calcium, protein, and pro-biotics for strong bones, a flat tummy, and gorgeous hair, skin, and nails. Coconut and almond yogurt are great options for vegans.

16 Pumpkin Puree

Pumpkin promotes healthy lungs and eyes and contains potassium, fiber, and vitamins A, B3, B5, B6, and C.

17 Sweet Potato Puree

Sweet potatoes are packed with fiber and contain loads of vitamins A and C, which promote beautiful skin and boost immunity.

18 Maple Syrup

This sap from the maple tree contains natural acids, calcium, potassium, and trace amounts of thiamin, magnesium, and riboflavin.

TOO MUCH SWEETNESS

Fruits add natural sweetness to juices, but they can also add a ton of sugar. Adding too many fruits can easily turn your healthy drink into a high-sugar dessert that can spike blood insulin levels. In fact, a tall glass of fruit juice can pack around 50 grams of the sweet stuff—more than twice the daily recommendation for women by the American Heart Association, and more than a full day's worth for men. The recipes in this book are Clean Green–approved to be low in sugar, but if you're experimenting (love that!), enjoy fruits in moderation and see that vegetables make up the bulk of your juices.

NOTE: Every juice and smoothie in this book has been sweetly balanced with your svelte figure in mind. You're already sweet enough, naturally! But if you must add sweeteners, go for these.

Agave

Agave may be higher in calories than sugar, but it is also sweeter, meaning you can use less. It also has a lower glycemic index, which helps maintain blood sugar levels.

Honey

Gotta totally love those hard-working bees! Honey boosts antioxidant levels in our blood, is filled with anti-cancer phytonutrients, and can strengthen your immune system. Look for raw or Grade-A honey, honey!

Molasses

Noted by my professor at Columbia University as the most nutrient-laden sweetener available, this sugarcane syrup contains manganese, iron, copper, and potassium.

Stevia

Stevia is a plant-derived, zero-calorie sweetener that is 250 times sweeter than sugar. It's a great choice for anyone looking to cut back on sugar or artificial sweeteners.

♥FROZEN
BANANA LOVE

The "skinny" on my frozen banana obsession:

If I learned one thing from my protein-workout-smoothie-addicted ex-boyfriend, it was that frozen bananas are a must. He made sure he always had a dozen or so in his freezer at any given time. So at the beginning of every week, grab a bunch of semi-ripe bananas at the market, and read on to learn how to store them for everyday smoothie perfection. And check out my fancy pictoral for you. Ooh la la!

1 Carefully unpeel the banana, so it stays intact for precise measuring. Discard the peel. (A frozen banana with the peel on is a nightmare to work with!)

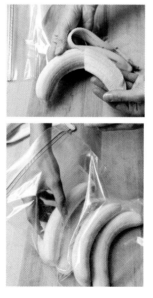

2 Place up to six peeled bananas into a resealable plastic freezer bag. Remove the air from the bag and seal tightly.

3 Keeping the bananas intact, carefully place the bag into your freezer; keep frozen for up to a few months. When you're ready to blend, remove the bag from the freezer and grab the amount of bananas needed. Break in half before placing into a blender. Immediately place the remaining frozen bananas back into the freezer.

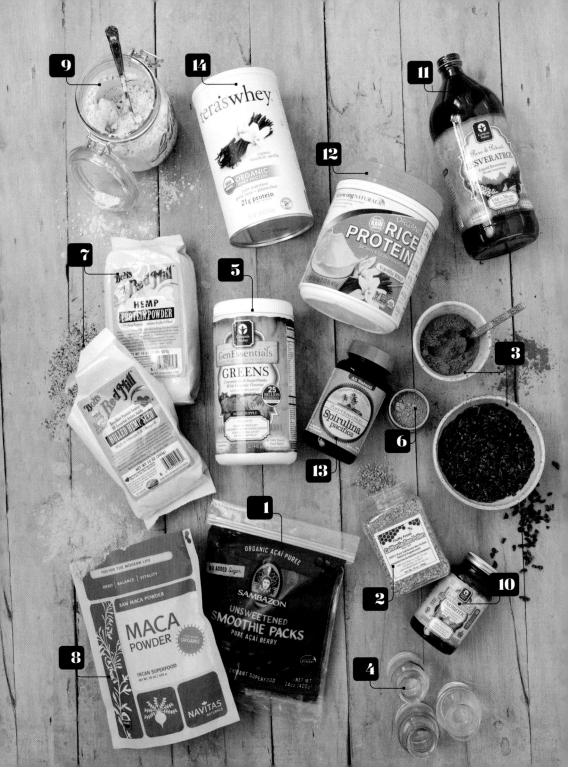

NATURAL SUPER-BOOSTERS

These ingredients can supercharge your Clean Green body, adding a boost of energy, protein, or even immunity—naturally.

BOOSTERS

1 Açai Berries
2 Bee Pollen
3 Dark Cocoa Powder & Cacao Nibs
4 Flaxseed Oil
5 Green Superfood
6 Green Tea Powder (Matcha)
7 Hemp Protein Powder & Hemp Seed
8 Maca Root Powder
9 Pea Protein Powder
10 Probiotics
11 Resveratrol
12 Rice Protein Powder
13 Spirulina
14 Whey Protein Powder

Açai Berries

These Brazilian super-boosters are now commonly found in the frozen section of health food stores. The berries are packed with anthocyanins and flavonoids, which are powerful antioxidants that may help aid in the prevention of cancer and the boosting of skin health. Consuming berries like açai may help fight aging by fighting free radicals (unstable atoms that can damage cells) in the body. Açai berries may also reduce cholesterol and blood pressure, thanks to their plant sterols, and may improve weight loss due to their high fiber content. These berries are delicious in your A.M. smoothies and best paired with coconut water and spinach. Superpowers!

41

2 Bee Pollen

A holistic remedy, bee pollen contains vitamins, minerals, carbohydrates, lipids, protein, and a massive amount of amino acids. It may help the digestive system, boost the immune system, support the cardiovascular system, and aid in prostate and infertility problems.

3 Dark Cocoa Powder and Cacao Nibs

Naturally packed with antioxidants, cocoa may aid in lowering cholesterol and blood pressure, which can lead to a healthier heart. Cocoa/cacao may also help to improve circulation and release feel-good chemicals, such as serotonin and endorphins. It contains essential fats and minerals, including calcium, magnesium, sulfur, zinc, and iron. Studies even show that chocolate can mimic the same happy feelings as kissing. Um, hello chocolate make-out session!

4 Flaxseed Oil

It's one of my big sister's favorite oils to add to her morning smoothies. Also known as linseed oil, flax oil is full of omega-3 fatty acids, alpha-linolenic acid (which may help boost immunity), and vitamin E. I like to add one teaspoon to some of my blended beauties to reap all these bennies.

5 Green Superfood Powder

Green superfood is bursting with vitamins A, C, and K; fiber; protein; thiamin; riboflavin; niacin; and omegas-3, -6 and -9. Plant sources include wheat grass, alfalfa grass, parsley, barley grass, oat grass, and spinach. There are many green powders on the market, but I like Energy Green SuperFood by Amazing Grass and Genesis Today's GenEssentials Greens.

6 Green Tea Powder (Matcha)

Matcha, or green tea powder, may aid in the prevention of cancer and can be used as a fat burner. Green tea contains a large amount of vitamins, minerals, antioxidants, and amino acids, and may help boost metabolism. It also has relaxing qualities (very Zen!), helps lower blood sugar and cholesterol, and can naturally detoxify the body. Check out Ito En for a great selection of teas/powders.

7 Hemp Protein Powder and Hemp Seed

A nutty and earthy powder or ground meal, hemp is a complete protein (meaning it contains all nine essential amino acids) that's also rich in iron, magnesium, and omega-3s, which can help prevent heart disease, dementia, and inflammation. Hemp also helps to repair and develop lean body mass. I've always been a fan of Bob's Redmill.

8 Maca Root Powder

Maca, a tuber grown in the Andes Mountains of Peru, may help improve the libido (wink, wink), enhance your mood, lower stress, help ease tension, and increase energy. It has also been used in holistic medicine as a pain reliever. Give it a try! Just sprinkle in a little and see if it does wonders for you, too.

DAILY PROTEIN NEEDS

There is no one-size-fits-all protein requirement. The recommended daily allowance for protein by the Centers for Disease Control and Prevention is 46g for women ages 19-70. However studies show that increased protein consumption (between 20 and 25 percent of total calories) can reduce the risk of heart disease, if the extra protein replaces refined carbohydrates, like white bread and sugary drinks.

9 Pea Protein Powder

My favorite vegan protein is high in lysine content; it may help lower cholesterol and promote a healthy immune system. Pea protein also helps aid in muscle recovery and contains antioxidants and anti-inflammatory agents. I like Vega and Growing Naturals brands.

10 Probiotics

Probiotics have been shown to aid digestion and boost the immune system. I purchase probiotics like acidophilus as capsules and prefer to sprinkle one or two into my smoothies as needed. They are virtually impossible to detect in any beverage. Or you can opt for yogurt or a liquid acidophilus product. I've been drinking these live-active cultures for years; they help keep your immunity up and your digestive system happy.

11 Resveratrol

Also referred to as the "fountain of youth," resveratrol—with its unique blend of seven plant sources—contains white, red, and Concord grape juices as the delicious base flavor. The Genesis Today brand combines resveratrol with Japanese knotweed extract, grapeseed and grape skin extract, aloe vera powder, and red wine extract—all without the hangover! Of course, if you prefer a glass of red wine, that also has anti-aging properties! Cheers! Enjoy life's greatest pleasures.

12 Rice Protein Powder

This vegan protein is isolated from carbs in rice and has a mild flavor. It is commonly combined with pea protein. Rice protein is gluten-free, hypoallergenic, and provides essential amino acids and fiber. Growing Naturals makes a delightful-tasting rice protein powder that blends beautifully into smoothies.

13 Spirulina

Spirulina, how do I love thee? Let me count the ways. This blue-green algae is rich in protein, vitamins, minerals, carotenoids, and antioxidants that fight off free radicals. It's also rich in beta-carotene, which may aid in the prevention of cancer and helps prevent aging (sounds fabulous!). This superb organic source of vitamin B12 may help decrease bad cholesterol, lower blood pressure, prevent infection, and naturally cleanse your system. Spirulina may also increase stamina (perfect for the gym and bedroom!) and help build sexy, lean muscle mass. Plus, it is a compete protein. Sounds like the most incredible superfood out there, right? Trust me, you will be a spirulina-addict, too. And yes, you will see mentions of this superfood numerous times throughout this book. I am a superfan! Look for powdered varieties in your local health food store. I prefer Pure Hawaiian Spirulina Pacifica by Nutrex.

14 Whey Protein Powder*

A byproduct of cheese production, whey protein promotes muscle growth, contains essential amino acids, and may have anti-cancer and anti-inflammatory properties. It may also help you lose weight, reduce high cholesterol and asthma symptoms, and lower blood pressure. *Contains dairy.*

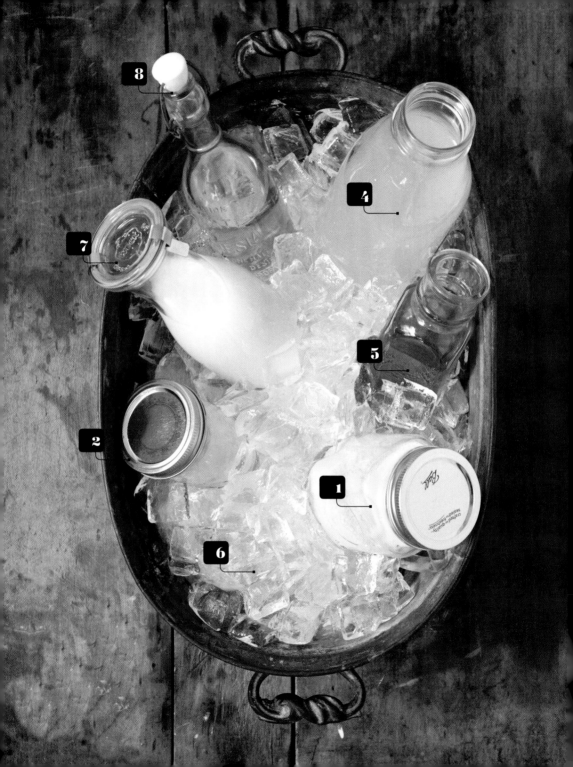

"If you want gorgeous, glowing skin and no dimples on that bum, drink more water! It's free." -CK

LIQUID GOLD

You'll notice that I'm not a fan of processed, sweetened juices. Why? Because they are huge contributors to obesity and other diseases in the U.S., and I refuse to allow you to chug excess calories. The only juices that you will be drinking are clean, green, fresh juices, directly from your juicer. When adding liquids to your blender for smoothies, I recommend the following options:

LIQUID GOLD

1 Almond Milk
2 Almond & Coconut Milk Blend
3 Coconut Milk Drink (not pictured)
4 Coconut Water
5 Green Tea
6 Ice
7 Rice Milk
8 Water

1 Almond Milk (Unsweetened)

At only 45 calories per cup, this choice is superior to any other. We've tried and tested every kind of milk out there, and unsweetened almond milk reigns supreme! Filled with vitamins D and E, phosphorus, and calcium, it can also promote beautiful hair, skin, and nails.

LUSTING FOR LEMON WATER

Health professionals hold lemon water in high regard for its numerous health benefits. Packed with vitamin C, a glass of lemon water each morning can help flush the body of toxins, boost your immune system, and even freshen your breath. For the best cleansing benefits, squeeze half of a big, juicy lemon—organic if possible—in a tall glass of lukewarm water. Why warm? Boiling water can destroy some of the fresh lemon's natural enzymes, while ice-cold water can hinder the digestive benefits. So there you go, Goldilocks: Lukewarm is *juuust* right.

2 Almond & Coconut Milk Blend (Unsweetened)

Created by Almond Breeze, this creamy, delicious, and nutrient-dense blend is a great nondairy choice to add richness and body to any recipe. Full of vitamins D and E and calcium, this beverage is one of the most frequently used liquids in the book.

3 Coconut Milk Drink (Unsweetened)

Note: This is not the same as canned whole coconut milk. This "coconut milk beverage" is lighter and found in the refrigerated section of most supermarkets. Great brands include Almond Breeze, So Delicious, Coconut Dream, and Silk. The creamy liquid from the meat of the coconut contains lauric acid, a medium-chain fatty acid also found in mother's milk, and is often enriched with good stuff like vitamins A, B12, and D; folate; iron; selenium; and magnesium.

4 Coconut Water

Lower in calories than fruit juices and naturally abundant in potassium and electrolytes, this is a great substitute for sugary energy drinks. And it contains natural magnesium and calcium. But beware: Some brands can also contain a large amount of sugar, so be sure to read the label.

48

5 **Green Tea** (Unsweetened)

Studies show green tea leaves can help aid weight loss and regulate blood sugar. They are full of antioxidants and anti-inflammatory and anti-cancer agents. Green tea is also rich in flavonoids, helps prevent heart disease, and promotes beautiful skin. My absolute favorites are Ito En's Teas' Tea; matcha green tea powder; and genmaicha, a Japanese toasted brown-rice tea.

6 **Ice**

At zero calories, ice adds waist-friendly volume to your smoothies. Herbal ice cubes are one of my favorite ways to preserve herbs and give smoothies a kick. After rinsing and drying, coarsely chop herbs. Fill an ice cube tray with generous pinches of the aromatic goodness and top with water (adding water first tends to leave the herbs floating).

7 **Rice Milk**

Rice milk has a much sweeter and lighter body than almond milk. If you like a bit of texture or a sweet finish, go for rice milk. Rice milk can be high in carbs, calories, and sugar, though, so be sure to check the label.

8 **Water**

The obvious zero-calorie choice, water adds volume to your smoothies and aids with satiety. The best part? It's free!

EQUIP ME

So what kind of investment are you going to have to make on this journey to reclaim your health and waistline? Well, let's just say it's a fraction of what your Louboutin heels or that Minkoff purse costs. These tools will last you years and years, even hundreds of cups later. Invest in your wellness.

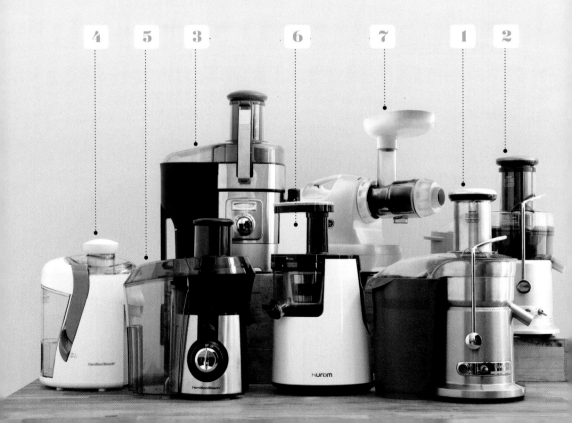

This is a collection of blenders and juicers that I have thoroughly tested for **a**) **performance, b**) **ease of use, c**) **cost,** and **d**) **quality.** There are hundreds of varieties to choose from, so I advise you to shop around, test, explore, and select what works best for your Clean Green lifestyle.

JUICERS

1 Breville Juice Fountain Elite 800JEXL ($300) *Centrifugal

One of Breville's most popular juicers, this 1,000-watt workhorse is renowned for both its power and ease to clean. I've personally used a Breville juicer for the past six years and can attest it's a breeze to clean. It works well for the everyday household and includes a one-year limited warranty.

2 Breville Juice Fountain Plus JE98XL ($150) *Centrifugal

My very first juicer, this is a wonderful beginner's machine or for someone on a budget. It's simple to use and clean, and it stores easily in your kitchen. A simple choice for a starter juicer, or as a gift for a friend that's just getting into Clean Green living.

3 Cuisinart Juice Extractor CJE-1000 ($150) *Centrifugal

Right in the middle of our juicer price range, this 1,000-watt juicer is a family favorite. It doesn't just look great: With a five-speed control dial, adjustable flow spout, and super-quiet motor, this is a great piece of equipment to have in the kitchen.

4 Hamilton Beach HealthSmart Juice Extractor ($40) *Centrifugal

Small but mighty, this 400-watt juicer is great for a beginner on a budget. You're going to have to cut up your veggies a bit to fit into the small opening, but it's great for anybody who has limited room in their kitchen and wants to start juicing without upgrading to total-pro level.

TIPS FOR CLEAN-ING YOUR JUICER

- **Clean your juicer right away**. Save time and protect your health by cleaning your tools as soon as you can after juicing. Fresh juice and pulp rinses easily, and any residue left on the juicer is a breeding ground for germs.

- **Line the pulp bin**. Lining the pulp chamber with a biodegradable bag makes cleanup a cinch. The pulp can be transferred into a compost bin, saved for baking, or put directly in the garbage.

- **Use hot water**. I like to fill the sink with hot, soapy water so all the removable parts of the juicer get a quick soak. (Consult your manufacturer's directions before putting anything in the dishwasher.)

- **Scrub the juicing screen**. The juicing screen or sieve can be the trickiest part of the juicer to clean. I recommend investing in a good scrubber, or even a toothbrush can also help get into the nooks and crannies.

5 Hamilton Beach Big Mouth Pro Juice Extractor ($80) *Centrifugal

A great starter juicer for someone looking to dive into the Clean Green life, this is an easy-to-assemble juicer with high horsepower and a wide flute; you'll be sipping your juice in no time! Easy cleanup is a bonus, too.

6 Hurom Premium Slow Juicer & Smoothie Maker HH ($400) *Masticating

If you have money to invest, go for this Hurom. It's a great option, since the slow masticating processing keeps your juice from oxidizing as quickly, and that means more vital nutrients! The model is absolutely sleek and stylish, too! I use this one daily and *love* it.

7 Omega 8004 Nutrition Center Juicer ($260) *Masticating

This Omega Nutrition Center Juicer is a masticating-style juice extractor. Juicing at a low speed reduces heat buildup, which retains more enzymes and nutrients. If you're nervous about the price, just know that it does more than just juice: You can also create baby food purees, and grind nut butters with the Omega.

For more on the difference between centrifugal and masticating juicers, see page 14.

1 Cuisinart PowerEdge 1,000-Watt Blender ($200)

If you're looking for an easy-to-use, versatile blender that's great for the family, this baby delivers. It has preset options such as "pulse," "ice crush," and of course, "smoothie." This blender also looks as good as it performs. The blender is straightforward, so you can quickly use and clean it before heading out the door. Cuisinart has a gorgeous collection of high-quality blenders that look beautiful in your kitchen.

2 KitchenAid 5-Speed Diamond Blender ($150)

This is the perfect blender to give to a friend or the parents. I purchased this for my mom and dad last Christmas, and they absolutely love it! It has the power to mix, chop, and stir all of their recipes. KitchenAid now makes their appliances in several shades of pink, donating part of the proceeds to the Susan G. Komen's Cook for the Cure to raise money and awareness for the fight against breast cancer. If you're into blending for a cause, check out their line of do-good appliances.

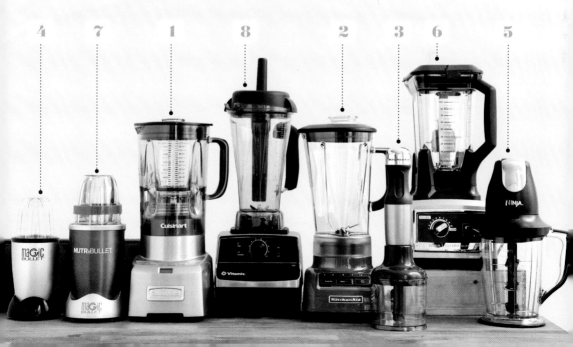

BLEND LIKE A PRO

- **Add liquids first.** It's easier on the blender and gets things moving faster.

- **Start at the lowest speed.** Wait a few seconds, or until the big pieces of fruit begin to break down, before turning up the speed. Going full throttle right away can create air bubbles and cause your blender to shake.

- **Play with liquid quantities.** For a thick, spoonable smoothie, use less liquid than dictated by the recipe.

3 KitchenAid 5-Speed Hand Blender ($130)

If you travel a lot, want a quick blend at the office, or love something lightweight and easy to clean, this hand blender will work for your busy lifestyle. It's easy to clean, has simple features, and includes a BPA-free cup. This immersion blender is also great for finishing off soup, sauces, and purees. Plus, its handheld size takes up little space in a small cupboard or drawer.

4 Magic Bullet ($100)

The Magic Bullet is an affordable new blending tool that has changed the game. This brilliantly updated model is a small, handheld, portable device that makes blending a breeze. From chopping onions to grating cheese or making Clean Green smoothies, the Magic Bullet blends quickly and efficiently. Cleanup is also much easier than most full-scale blenders. Note: The Magic Bullet "tall cup" is smaller than a regular blender, so you may need to cut recipes in half.

5 Ninja Master Prep ($90)

The Ninja Master Prep is a great, compact choice for an individual with limited kitchen space and who loves to blend and run. This Ninja Master Prep crushes ice well and blends two times faster than most blenders. It's also easy to clean.

6 Ninja Ultima Blender244 ($200)

I've used this blender for the past year, and it performs properly. Not only does it crush ice and blend up your fruits and veggies quickly at controlled levels, it's also simple to clean and boasts extra safety features. If you're into what the pros use, check out this professional high-speed blender. It has the horsepower, torque, and engineered blade speed to create chef-inspired results at home.

7 NutriBullet ($120)

The handheld, travel-friendly NutriBullet was designed to blend greens, seeds, beets, ginger, and even wheat grass! It allows you to mix super nutrient-packed drinks that taste great and take only seconds to make. Easy to clean, portable, and affordable, the NutriBullet has helped several of my friends shed pounds using my Clean Green recipes. They love chatting and gushing about this blender; it's got dedicated fans. Note: The NutriBullet "tall cup" is smaller than a regular blender, so you may need to cut recipes in half.

8 Vitamix 5200 ($450)

Noted as the "Mercedes-Benz of blenders," the Vitamix stuns in sleek brushed stainless steel and has a seven-year warranty, high-speed settings, variable speed control, and an amazing patented tamper that helps blend even the toughest frozen fruit. You can also make soups, purees, sauces, and frozen desserts. This blender is surely an investment, but it's worth its weight in green gold.

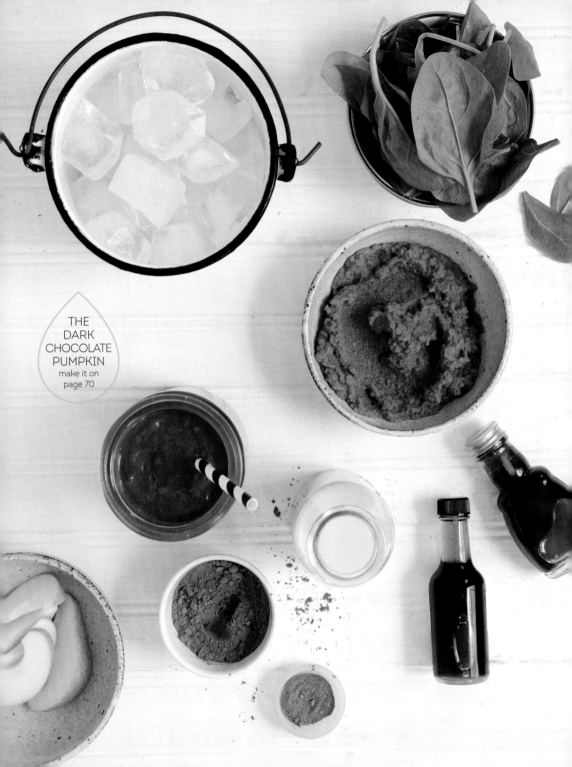

THE
DARK
CHOCOLATE
PUMPKIN
make it on
page 70

3

Cleansing Juices & Smoothies

(All 130 Calories or Less Per Serving!)

YOU DESERVE TO feel your very best every day. Although we don't always have time to bust out a plate of fruit and cheese with a side of steamed vegetables and quinoa at every meal, we can certainly make time to juice, blend, and cleanse. I've customized these quick "cleansing" recipes for you to reset your body and mind anytime. Enjoy—food is love.

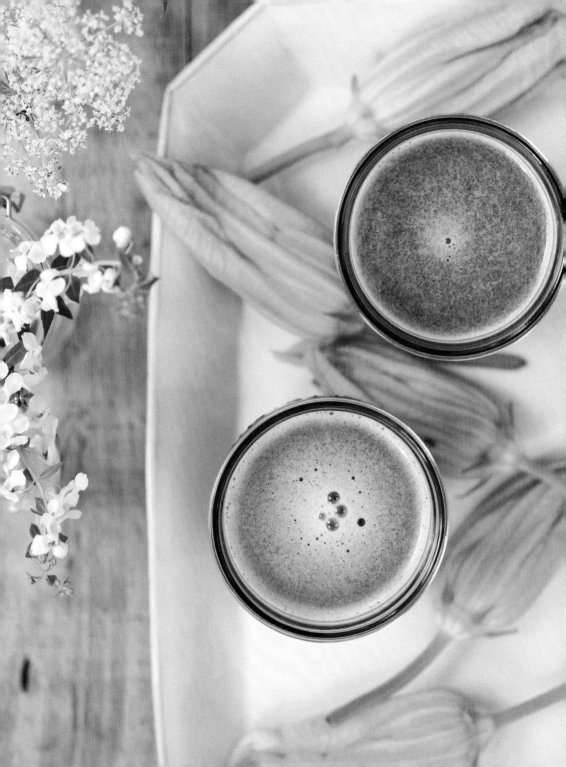

THE CUCUMBER-HONEYDEW MELON

JUICE › CUCUMBER, KALE, HONEYDEW MELON

1 **medium cucumber**

2 **cups kale**

¾ **cup honeydew melon**

Add all ingredients into a juicer and juice.

Cucumber and melon: Sounds like that lotion you used to smear all over your body circa 1992, right? It's actually a delicious combination, perfect for cooling and hydrating, or just to feel amazing.

SERVES 2 ▶ **PER SERVING** 100 CALORIES | 0 G FAT | 4 G PROTEIN | 21 G CARBOHYDRATES | 5 G FIBER | 16 G SUGAR | 500 MG POTASSIUM | 60% DV VITAMIN C | 10% DV IRON

Importance of Juicing Order

PROCESS THE HEARTY fruits and veggies first. Second, add leafy greens and herbs. Third, add more fleshy/watery fruits and vegetables to "wash out" the juicer. This makes cleanup easier—and will leave no precious greens behind!

THE BEETROOT BLEND

JUICE ▸ BEET, BABY SPINACH, APPLE

1 large beet, scrubbed, halved

4 cups baby spinach

½ Fuji apple, cored

Add all ingredients into a juicer and juice.

This easy-to-whip-up combination is quick for any morning juice to go. I love adding a dash of nutmeg, cinnamon, or pumpkin spice for some delightful essence in the A.M. Mmm, it's like fall every day!

SERVES 2 ▸ **PER SERVING** 90 CALORIES | 0 G FAT | 5 G PROTEIN | 19 G CARBOHYDRATES | 0 G FIBER | 18 G SUGAR | 69 MG POTASSIUM | 25% DV IRON | 50% DV FOLATE

THE SUPER BEET & KALE CLEANSER

JUICE ▸ BEET, KALE, CUCUMBER

2 medium beets, scrubbed, halved

4 cups kale

1 medium cucumber

¼ lemon

¼ teaspoon cinnamon

Add all ingredients into a juicer and juice. Pour into glass and whisk in cinnamon.

Turn up the beet! This "think pink" juice will get you feeling good after the first sip! Kale and cucumber are the perfect complements to this deep pink root, and a dash of cinnamon adds spice (not to mention some pretty fabulous health benefits). Cheers to you!

SERVES 2 ▸ **PER SERVING** 90 CALORIES | 1.5 G FAT | 8 G PROTEIN | 17 G CARBOHYDRATES | 0 G FIBER | 7 G SUGAR | 250 MG OMEGA-3 | 1,070 MG POTASSIUM | 35% DV FOLATE

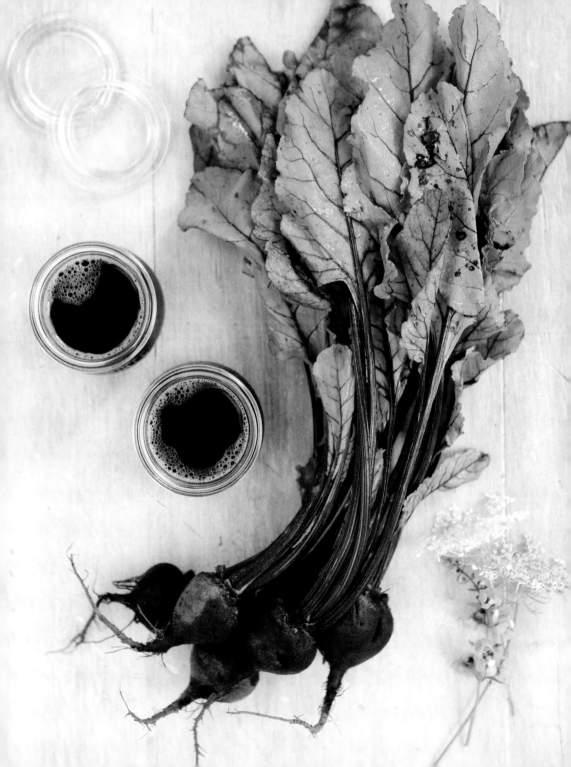

THE STRAWBERRY-
WATERMELON REFRESHER

SMOOTHIE 〉 STRAWBERRY, WATERMELON, BASIL

1 **cup unsweetened almond milk**

1 **cup frozen strawberries**

1 **cup watermelon**

1 **tablespoon fresh basil**

1 **cup ice**

Add ingredients into a blender and blend until smooth.

No need for expensive spa splurges. This "spa-like" combination of strawberries, watermelon, and basil can be blended right in your own kitchen. Invite the girls over, hire a few manicurists, whip up a few of these babies, and you've got the spa-weekend-in treatment. Cheers!

SERVES 2 ▶ **PER SERVING** 70 CALORIES ⋮ 15 G FAT ⋮
1 G PROTEIN ⋮ 15 G CARBOHYDRATES ⋮ 3 G FIBER ⋮ 10 G SUGAR ⋮
60% DV VITAMIN C ⋮ 10% DV VITAMIN D ⋮ 25% DV VITAMIN E

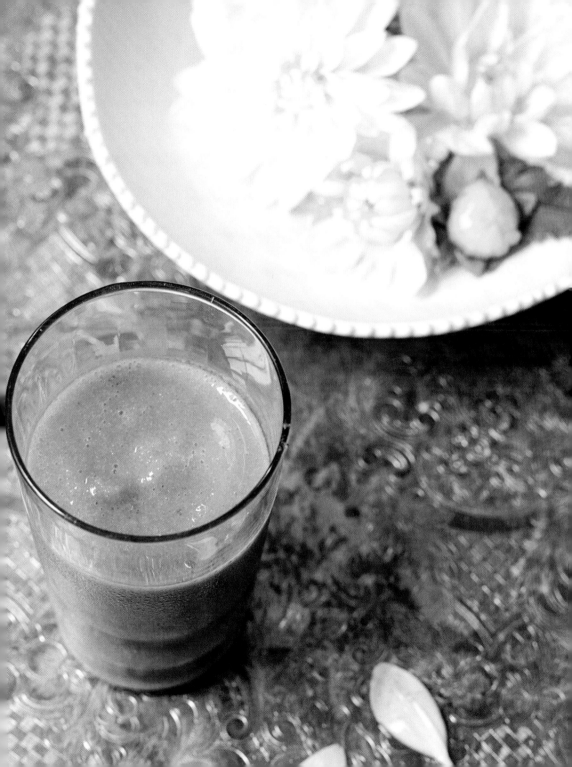

THE JUICY WATERMELON

JUICE › WATERMELON, BABY SPINACH, KALE, CUCUMBER

4 cups watermelon

1 cup baby spinach

1 cup kale

1 large cucumber

Add all ingredients into a juicer and juice.

Did you know that watermelon is full of natural electrolytes? Yes; it's just like that "vitamin-enhanced" water you blow all of your savings on. If only produce could do all of the talking. Check out this naturally hydrating juice that's also low in calories and full of nutrients! No labels needed.

SERVES 2 ▶ **PER SERVING** 90 CALORIES | 1 G FAT | 4 G PROTEIN | 21 G CARBOHYDRATES | 0 G FIBER | 16 G SUGAR | 100% DV VITAMIN A | 110% DV VITAMIN C

THE CUCUMBER CLEANSER

JUICE › APPLE, KALE, CUCUMBER

1 Fuji apple, quartered

2 cups kale

1 large cucumber

Add all ingredients into a juicer and juice.

This simple three-ingredient blend is a great beginner's juice that anyone can try. With these fresh ingredients and cell-boosting results, you will look and feel like a million bucks after a few weeks.

SERVES 2 ▶ **PER SERVING** 70 CALORIES | 1 G FAT | 4 G PROTEIN | 15 G CARBOHYDRATES | 0 G FIBER | 10 G SUGAR | 120 MG OMEGA-3 | 130% DV VITAMIN A | 150% DV VITAMIN C

THE SOUR APPLE

JUICE ❯ ROMAINE, BABY SPINACH, APPLE, GINGER, LEMON

½–¾ head romaine lettuce

3 cups baby spinach

½ Fuji or Granny Smith apple

1 teaspoon fresh ginger (optional)

1 tablespoon lemon juice

Add all ingredients into a juicer and juice. Pour into glass, whisk in lemon juice, and serve immediately.

A little tart and a little sweet, this perfect combination of apple, romaine, baby spinach, ginger, and lemon will have you feeling super-cleansed and refreshed.

SERVES 1 ▶ **PER SERVING** 70 CALORIES ǀ 1 G FAT ǀ 5 G PROTEIN ǀ 15 G CARBOHYDRATES ǀ 0 G FIBER ǀ 12 G SUGAR ǀ 360 MG OMEGA-3 ǀ 30% DV IRON ǀ 110% DV FOLATE

THE DANDELION DETOX

SMOOTHIE ❯ DANDELION, PINEAPPLE

1 cup unsweetened almond milk

2 cups dandelion greens

1 cup pineapple

1 cup ice

Add ingredients into a blender and blend until smooth.

Dandelion, with its bitter taste, can be naturally softened by sweet, sweet, pineapple. This four-ingredient smoothie is a perfect refresher on the weekends and a delicious way to savor the benefits of dandelion greens. Yum!

SERVES 2 ▶ **PER SERVING** 90 CALORIES ǀ 2 G FAT ǀ 2 G PROTEIN ǀ 17 G CARBOHYDRATES ǀ 4 G FIBER ǀ 9 G SUGAR ǀ 400 MG POTASSIUM ǀ 20% DV CALCIUM ǀ 35% DV VITAMIN E

65

THE BLUEBERRY DETOX BLEND

SMOOTHIE › BLUEBERRY, BABY SPINACH, BANANA, SPIRULINA

2 cups coconut water

2 cups baby spinach

2 cups frozen blueberries

½ frozen banana

2 tablespoons spirulina

1 cup of ice (optional)

Add ingredients into a blender and blend until smooth.

One of my favorite ways to detox, this Blueberry Detox Blend will get you back to YOU again. I whip up this mix for a quick lunch when heading out the door to meetings or just before a workout. Trust me, you're not going to want to skip that addition of spirulina. It's the new—dare I say—super-drug.

SERVES 4 ▶ **PER SERVING** 90 CALORIES ⏐ 1 G FAT ⏐ 4 G PROTEIN ⏐ 18 G CARBOHYDRATES ⏐ 4 G FIBER ⏐ 11 G SUGAR ⏐ 440 MG POTASSIUM ⏐ 10% DV IRON

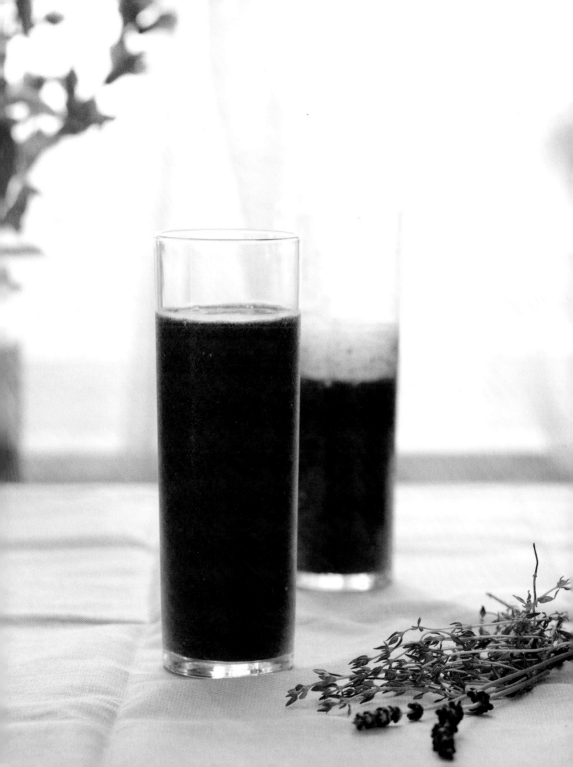

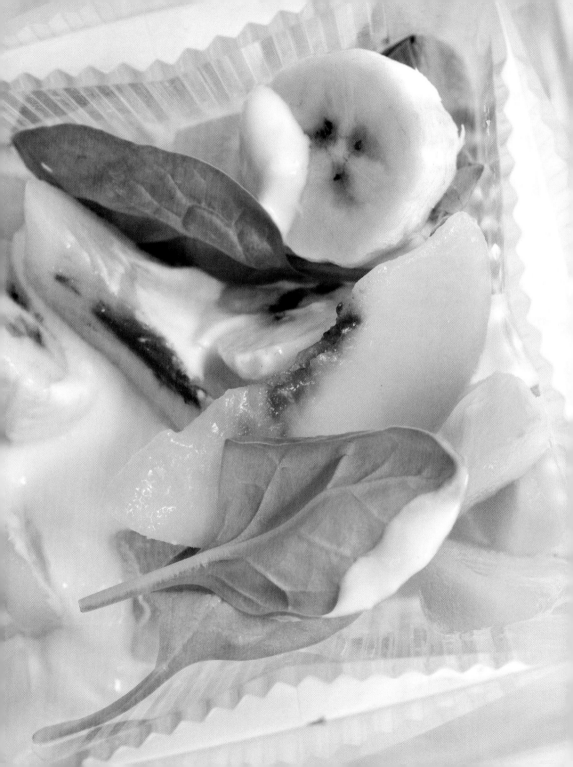

THE GREEN PEACHES AND CREAM

SMOOTHIE › BABY SPINACH, PEACH, BANANA, SPIRULINA

1¼ cups unsweetened
   almond milk

1 cup Greek or coconut
   yogurt

2 cups baby spinach

2 cups frozen peaches

½ frozen banana

1 tablespoon spirulina

Add ingredients into a
blender and blend until
smooth.

Peaches can have a mild-yet-tart flavor. Blend them
with some almond milk, coconut (or Greek) yogurt,
frozen banana, spinach, and Hawaiian spirulina.
You've just concocted the perfect Clean Green
smoothie to cleanse and keep up that immunity.

SERVES 2 ▶ **PER SERVING** 130 CALORIES | 2 G FAT |
4 G PROTEIN | 25 G CARBOHYDRATES | 2 G FIBER | 18 G SUGAR |
110% DV VITAMIN C | 15% DV CALCIUM | 15% DV VITAMIN D

THE DARK CHOCOLATE
PUMPKIN

1 cup unsweetened almond milk

1 cup organic pumpkin puree

3 cups baby spinach

½ Bartlett pear, cored

¼ frozen banana

2 tablespoons organic unsweetened cocoa powder

1 tablespoon maple syrup (optional, to taste)

¼ teaspoon pumpkin spice

1 cup ice

Add ingredients into a blender and blend until smooth.

Pumpkin and chocolate is a match made in heaven. The addition of fragrant Bartlett pears, a touch of maple syrup, and, of course, pumpkin spice, makes this drink downright decadent. Enjoy the indulgent ridiculousness and all of the natural nutritional benefits from this Clean Green smoothie, honey.

SERVES 4 ▶ **PER SERVING** 80 CALORIES | 2 G FAT | 3 G PROTEIN | 18 G CARBOHYDRATES | 7 G FIBER | 7 G SUGAR | 220% DV VITAMIN A | 20% DV VITAMIN E

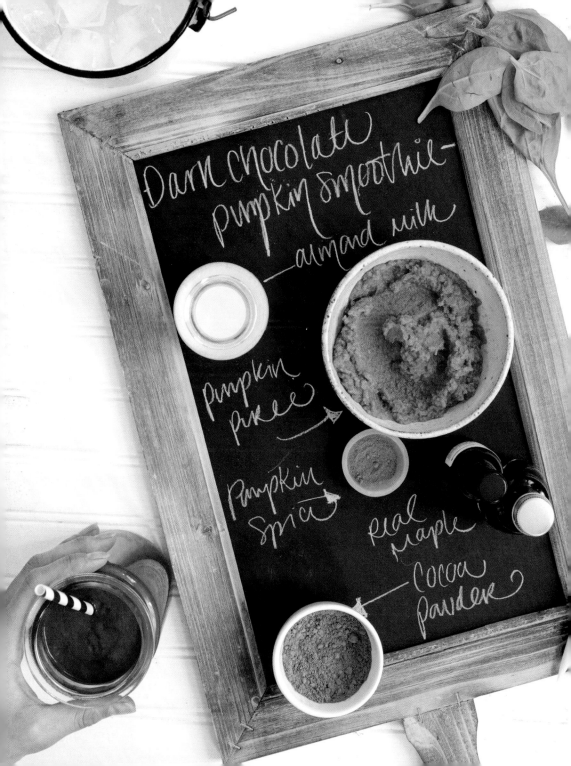

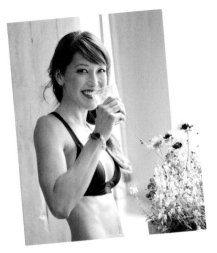

THE CHOCOLATE SKINNY "SHAKE"
SMOOTHIE › BABY SPINACH, BANANA, CHOCOLATE

1 **cup unsweetened coconut milk**

2 **cups baby spinach**

½ **frozen banana**

2 **tablespoons unsweetened cocoa powder**

1 **tablespoon green superfood**

1 **tablespoon pure maple syrup**

1 **cup ice**

Add ingredients into a blender and blend until smooth.

If you're anything like me, you love all things chocolate. But, alas, we can't always consume chocolate milkshakes and still fit into those teeny bikinis. Let's opt for this Chocolate Skinny "Shake," shall we? It satisfies and has some superfood kick to it. Go, you ninja, you.

SERVES 4 ▶ **PER SERVING** 120 CALORIES ⋮ 3.5 G FAT ⋮ 3 G PROTEIN ⋮ 24 G CARBOHYDRATES ⋮ 7 G FIBER ⋮ 11 G SUGAR ⋮ 50% DV VITAMIN A ⋮ 20% DV CALCIUM ⋮ 40% DV IRON

THE CUCUMBER HONEYDEW-MELON CLEANSER

SMOOTHIE › MELON, CUCUMBER, MINT

1 cup coconut water

1 cup honeydew melon

2 cucumbers

1 tablespoon fresh mint

1 cup ice

Add ingredients into a blender and blend until smooth.

This perfect blend of fresh mint, cucumber, honeydew melon, and coconut water will have you feeling clean, lean, and green. I love blending up this combo before hitting a yoga or meditation class in the afternoon. Talk about finding your inner "green." Reveal your true self.

SERVES 2 ▶ **PER SERVING** 60 CALORIES | 1 G FAT | 4 G PROTEIN | 11 G CARBOHYDRATES | 0 G FIBER | 7 G SUGAR | 140 MG OMEGA-3 | 610 MG POTASSIUM | 160% DV VITAMIN C

Chew Your Juice

SOUNDS CRAZY, RIGHT? Yet, chewing your green drink and swirling it in your mouth are important parts of the digestive process. That's because saliva contains the enzyme ptyalin, which helps break down food and speed up chemical reactions. A recent study by Purdue University confirmed a direct relationship between small particle size and increased nutrient uptake. In other words, the more you chew, the more nutrients your body can retain. Yummy!

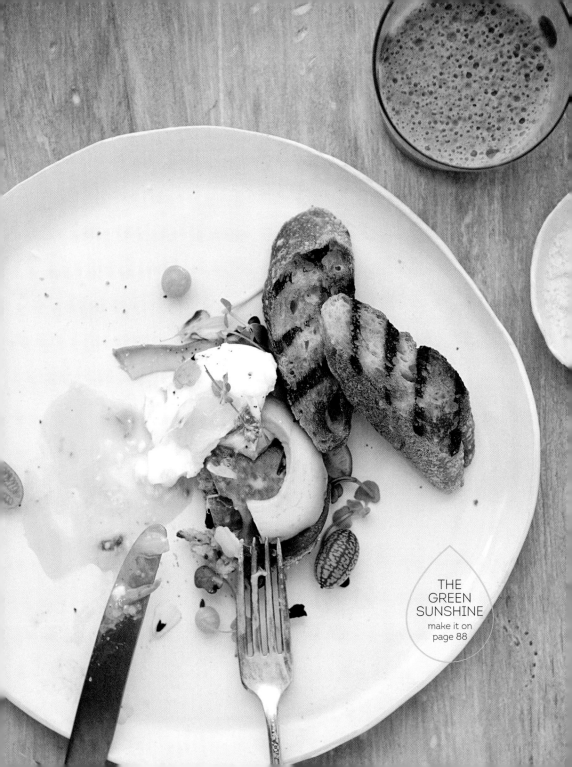

THE
GREEN
SUNSHINE
make it on
page 88

4

> "Be the kind of person you'd want to wake up next to."
> *– C.K.*

Morning Starter Juices & Smoothies

UPON WAKING, you should always feel like sunshine! Try these 10 delicious Clean Green ways to start the morning. If you're too stretched for time to make a smoothie in the A.M., prepare all of your frozen ingredients in a freezer bag the night before and just add the liquids and super-boosters the next day. Make it a priority to try these green drinks for a few weeks, and watch how energized you'll feel! Your friends and colleagues will notice a difference in your appearance, too. Reveal your true self. Glow green.

THE SWEET MELON
KALE ELIXIR

4 cups kale

1 cup honeydew melon

1 medium cucumber

1 tablespoon lemon juice

Add all ingredients into a juicer and juice. Pour into glass, whisk in lemon juice, and serve immediately.

With a hint of refreshing honeydew melon, cucumber, and our dear friend kale, this Clean Green juice is a sweet and hydrating way to nourish your beautiful body in the morning.

SERVES 1 ▶ **PER SERVING** 90 CALORIES | 1.5 G FAT | 7 G PROTEIN | 18 G CARBOHYDRATES | 0 G FIBER | 8 G SUGAR | 990 MG POTASSIUM | 270% DV VITAMIN A | 300% DV VITAMIN C

Clean Green FYI

JUICING ALONE cannot give you all of the nutrients you need in a day: The process of juicing extracts the produce pulp, which contains essential fiber and nutrients; plus you need other macronutrients like protein and healthy fats. So, make sure to eat a clean, protein-packed meal to balance out your day, and try adding a bit of the pulp back to your juice for optimal digestive health.

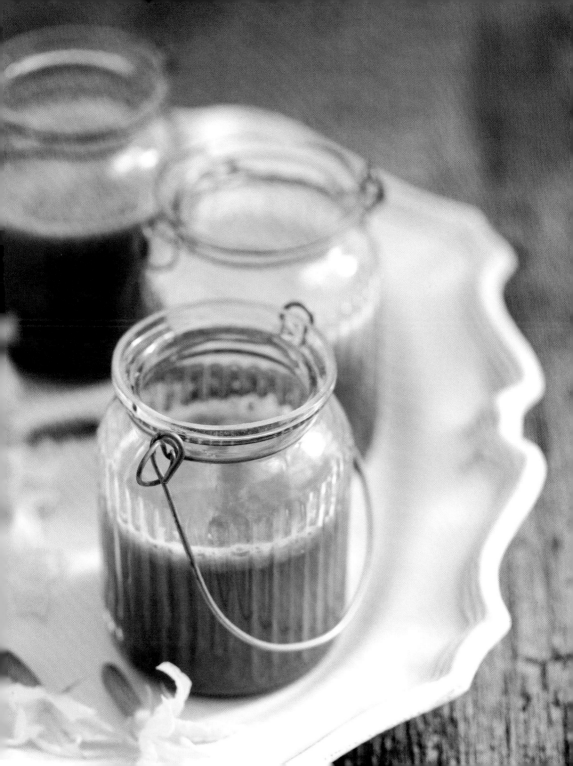

THE CINNAMON BEET

JUICE ▸ BABY SPINACH, KALE, BEET, CUCUMBER

2 cups baby spinach

1 cup kale

1 medium beet, scrubbed, halved

1 medium cucumber

¼ teaspoon cinnamon

Add all ingredients into a juicer and juice. Whisk in the cinnamon and serve.

Sweet, fragrant, cleansing, and good for you? You bet! This fresh juice will get you up and out of bed, and give your boring cup of joe a slap in the face.

SERVES 1 ▸ **PER SERVING** 80 CALORIES | 1 G FAT | 6 G PROTEIN | 14 G CARBOHYDRATES | 0 G FIBER | 8 G SUGAR | 870 MG POTASSIUM | 170% DV VITAMIN A | 20% DV CALCIUM | 30% DV FOLATE

THE BEETROOT-SUNSHINE BLEND

JUICE ▸ BABY SPINACH, BEET, CELERY, PEAR, LEMON

5 cups baby spinach

2 stalks celery

1 medium beet, scrubbed, quartered

¼ Bartlett pear, cored

¼ lemon, sliced

Add all ingredients into a juicer and juice.

Good morning, sunshine! Want to juice up something for you and your loved one in the A.M.? Try out this energizing combination of beets, pear, and a slice of lemon to wake up your cells and replenish your body.

SERVES 2 ▸ **PER SERVING** 70 CALORIES | 0 G FAT | 4 G PROTEIN | 13 G CARBOHYDRATES | 0 G FIBER | 11 G SUGAR | 90% DV VITAMIN A | 25% DV IRON | 25% DV FOLATE

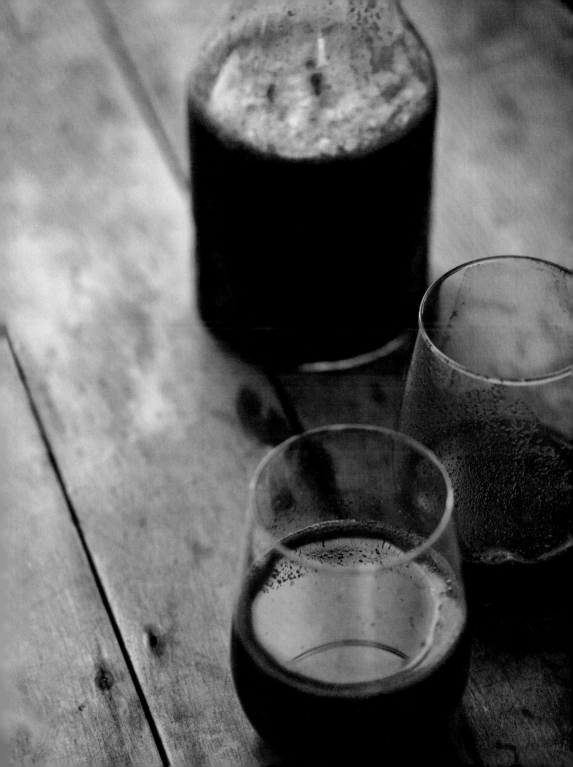

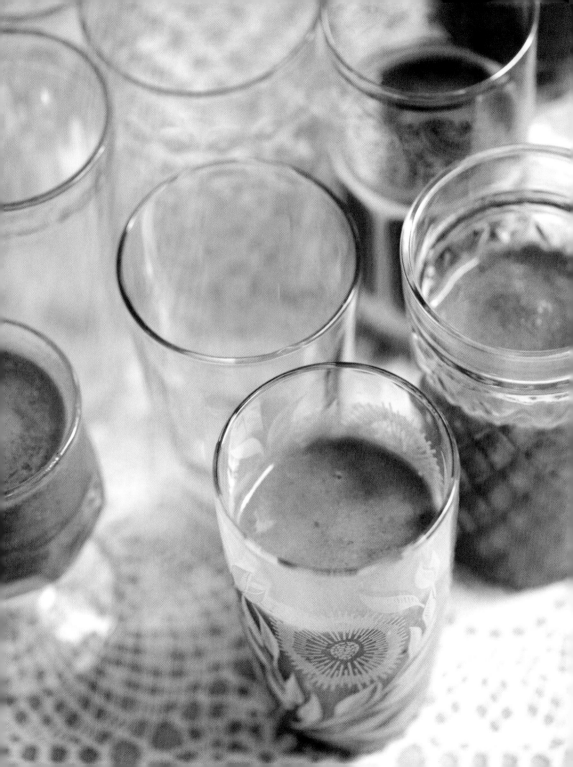

THE RASPBERRY MINT REFRESHER

SMOOTHIE ▸ RASPBERRY, BANANA, MINT, PROBIOTICS

1½ cups unsweetened
  almond milk

2 cups frozen
  raspberries

½ frozen banana

1 tablespoon fresh mint

1 teaspoon probiotics

1 cup ice

Add ingredients into a
blender and blend until
smooth.

This fresh and delicious smoothie will have you feeling like sunshine all day with its blend of raspberries, mint, and a touch of banana. Go for it, gorgeous!

SERVES 2 ▸ **PER SERVING** 100 CALORIES | 2.5 G FAT | 2 G PROTEIN |
22 G CARBOHYDRATES | 6 G FIBER | 8 G SUGAR | 15% DV CALCIUM |
20% DV VITAMIN D | 40% DV VITAMIN E

THE CHOCOLATE
MORNING WAKE-UP

1 **cup unsweetened almond milk**

1 **cup baby spinach**

1 **frozen banana**

2 **tablespoons unsweetened cocoa powder**

1 **tablespoon green superfood**

2 **tablespoons protein powder**

1 **cup ice**

Add ingredients into a blender and blend until smooth.

Chocolate does a body good! Just look at all of the benefits that cocoa powder and cacao nibs can bring into your Clean Green life: See page 42. Your taste buds can thank me later, hon.

SERVES 2 ▶ **PER SERVING** 150 CALORIES ⁞ 2.5 G FAT ⁞ 10 G PROTEIN ⁞ 23 G CARBOHYDRATES ⁞ 7 G FIBER ⁞ 8 G SUGAR ⁞ 25% DV CALCIUM ⁞ 50% DV IRON ⁞ 25% DV VITAMIN E

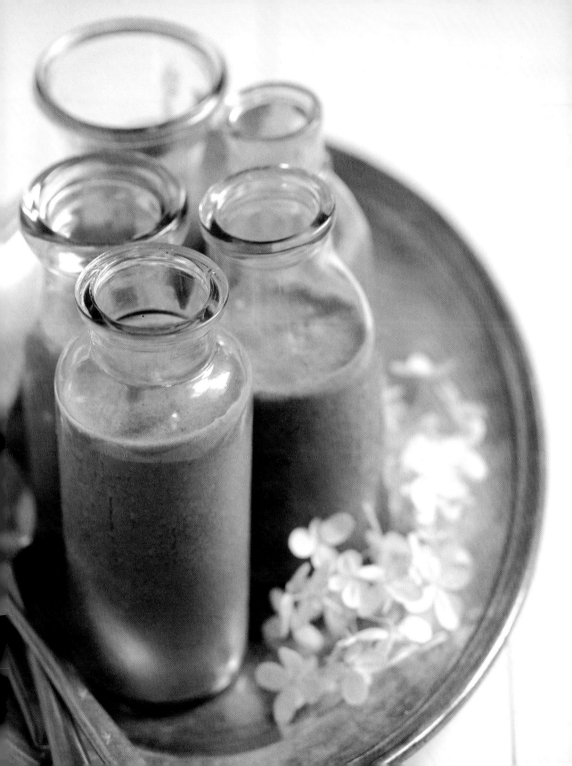

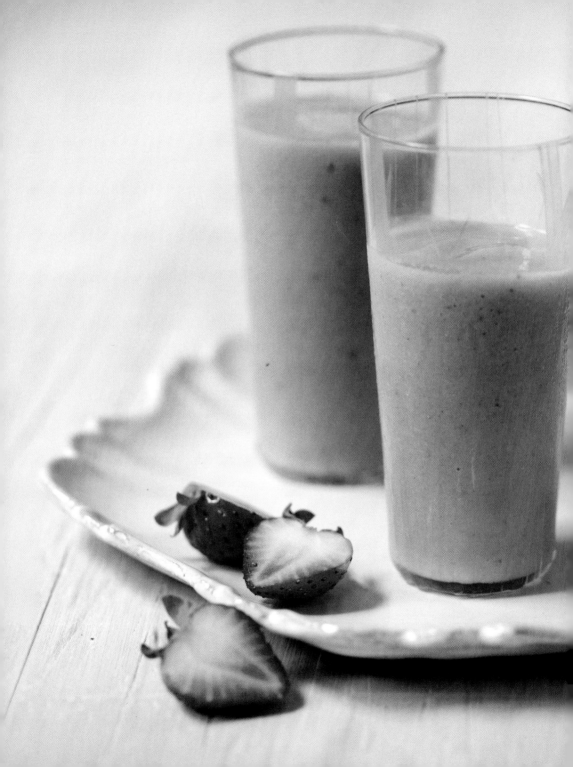

THE HAWAII FIVE-O

SMOOTHIE > PINEAPPLE, MANGO, COCONUT

1½ cups unsweetened almond milk

¾ cup pineapple

1 cup frozen mango

1 tablespoon shredded coconut

1 cup ice

Add ingredients into a blender and blend until smooth.

Pineapple, mango, and shredded coconut?! Aloha, Mister Hand! (My plug to *Fast Times at Ridgemont High*.) You'll be taken back to Honolulu in no time.

SERVES 4 ▶ **PER SERVING** 60 CALORIES ¦ 1.5 G FAT ¦ 1 G PROTEIN ¦ 13 G CARBOHYDRATES ¦ 2 G FIBER ¦ 10 G SUGAR ¦ 45% DV VITAMIN C ¦ 20% DV VITAMIN E

THE STRAWBERRY MANGO MORNING

SMOOTHIE > BABY SPINACH, STRAWBERRY, MANGO, PROTEIN POWDER

1¾ cups unsweetened coconut milk drink

1 cup baby spinach

1 cup frozen strawberries

1 cup frozen (or fresh) mango

4 tablespoons protein powder

1 cup ice

Add ingredients into a blender and blend until smooth.

Good morning, lovely! This recipe was developed to prevent inflammation, reduce wrinkles, and enhance lean-muscle building. Be beautiful and strong.

SERVES 4 ▶ **PER SERVING** 110 CALORIES ¦ 2 G FAT ¦ 6 G PROTEIN ¦ 16 G CARBOHYDRATES ¦ 3 G FIBER ¦ 12 G SUGAR ¦ 15% DV IRON ¦ 15% DV VITAMIN D

THE GREEN MATCHA TEA

SMOOTHIE › BABY SPINACH, BANANA, MATCHA, BEE POLLEN

1½ cups coconut water

2 cups baby spinach

1 frozen banana

2 teaspoons matcha green tea powder

1 teaspoon bee pollen

1 cup ice

Add ingredients into a blender and blend until smooth.

Wakie-wakie with this super-delicious smoothie, and head out for a meditation or yoga session. I highly recommend cleansing all areas of your life: mental, physical, and spiritual. Green tea will get you there.

SERVES 4 ▶ **PER SERVING** 70 CALORIES | 0 G FAT |
1 G PROTEIN | 17 G CARBOHYDRATES | 2 G FIBER | 9 G SUGAR |
410 MG POTASSIUM

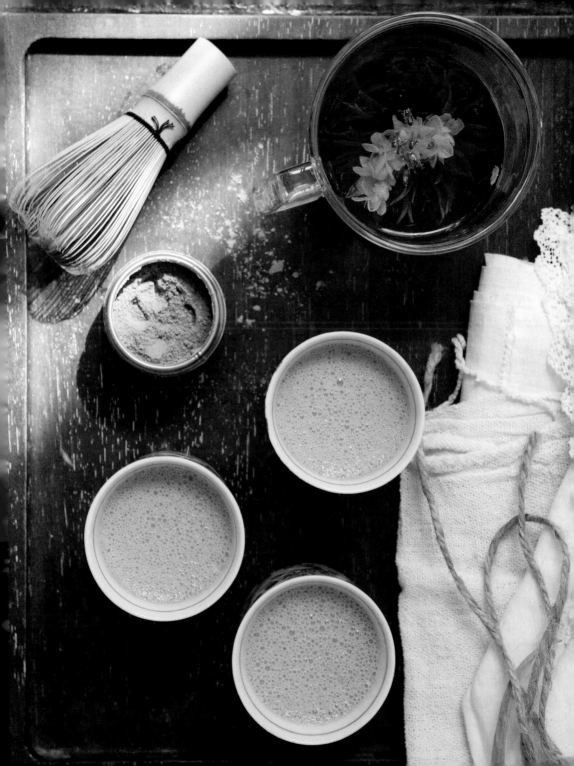

THE GREEN SUNSHINE

SMOOTHIE ❯ BABY SPINACH, BANANA, APPLE, GREEN SUPERFOOD

1 cup unsweetened almond milk

2 cups baby spinach

1 frozen banana

½ Fuji apple

1 tablespoon green superfood

1 tablespoon spirulina

1 cup ice

Add ingredients into a blender and blend until smooth.

Good morning, green sunshine! With this tasty green combination of baby spinach, spirulina, and green superfood, you are off to a sunny and beautiful morning! Enjoy and share the green glow love with your mate or a colleague at work.

SERVES 2 ▶ **PER SERVING** 140 CALORIES ⁞ 2 G FAT ⁞ 5 G PROTEIN ⁞ 27 G CARBOHYDRATES ⁞ 7 G FIBER ⁞ 12 G SUGAR ⁞ 510 MG POTASSIUM ⁞ 25% DV CALCIUM ⁞ 45% DV IRON

THE BREAKFAST BLEND

SMOOTHIE ❯ BABY SPINACH, BLUEBERRY, BANANA, GREEN SUPERFOOD

2 cups unsweetened almond milk

2 cups baby spinach

1½ cups frozen blueberries

1 frozen banana

¼ cup green superfood

1 teaspoon spirulina

1 cup ice

Add ingredients into a blender and blend until smooth.

Who needs Wheaties when you can drink the new gold standard of breakfast? This perfect blend is bursting with superfoods like blueberries, spinach, and spirulina.

SERVES 3 ▶ **PER SERVING** 130 CALORIES ⁞ 2.5 G FAT ⁞ 5 G PROTEIN ⁞ 24 G CARBOHYDRATES ⁞ 8 G FIBER ⁞ 9 G SUGAR ⁞ 150 MG OMEGA-3 ⁞ 70% DV IRON ⁞ 25% DV VITAMIN E

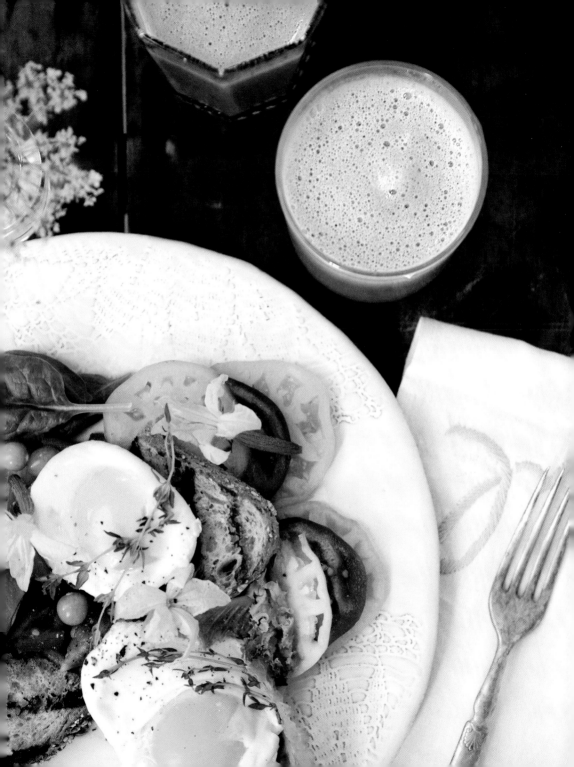

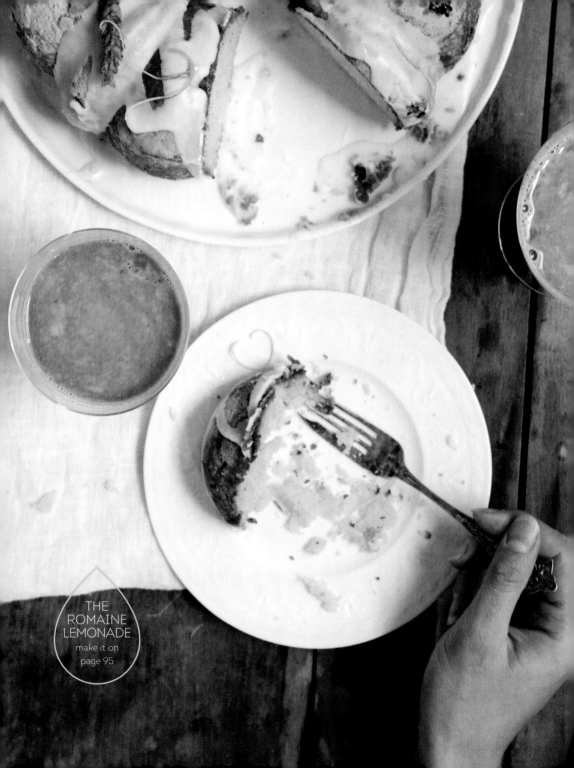

THE
ROMAINE
LEMONADE
make it on
page 95

5

Filling Juices & Smoothies

TEN TASTY WAYS to fill your tum, drink your greens, and get moving! Let's get semi-serious here: Filling fiber can improve all areas of your life. It can give you a flatter belly, lower cholesterol, easier digestion, a new boyfriend... Well, that last part I made up. But there are so many bennies. So take advantage with these high-fiber smoothies and surprisingly filling green juices.

THE KALE APPLE

JUICE > KALE, APPLE, CUCUMBER

4 cups kale

1 Fuji apple

1 large cucumber

¼ lemon (optional)

Add all ingredients into a juicer and juice.

With clean ingredients all around—apples, kale, and cucumber—you'll feel immediately recharged and revitalized by sipping this juice. For an extra touch of detox, add in one-quarter of a lemon.

SERVES 1-2 ▶ **PER SERVING** 100 CALORIES | 1.5 G FAT | 7 G PROTEIN | 20 G CARBOHYDRATES | 0 G FIBER | 10 G SUGAR | 240 MG OMEGA-3 | 920 MG POTASSIUM | 280% DV VITAMIN C

THE DANDELION GREEN PINEAPPLE

JUICE > PINEAPPLE, DANDELION, BABY SPINACH

1½ cups fresh pineapple

2 cups dandelion greens

2 cups baby spinach

1½ cups coconut water

Add all ingredients into a juicer and juice. Then whisk in coconut water to combine.

If you are finally up for the dandelion greens challenge, then this is your juice. Packed with antioxidants and potassium, this bitter green can also help to purify the blood and liver.

SERVES 2 ▶ **PER SERVING** 70 CALORIES | 0 G FAT | 2 G PROTEIN | 17 G CARBOHYDRATES | 0 G FIBER | 12 G SUGAR | 470 MG POTASSIUM | 90% DV VITAMIN A | 10% DV IRON

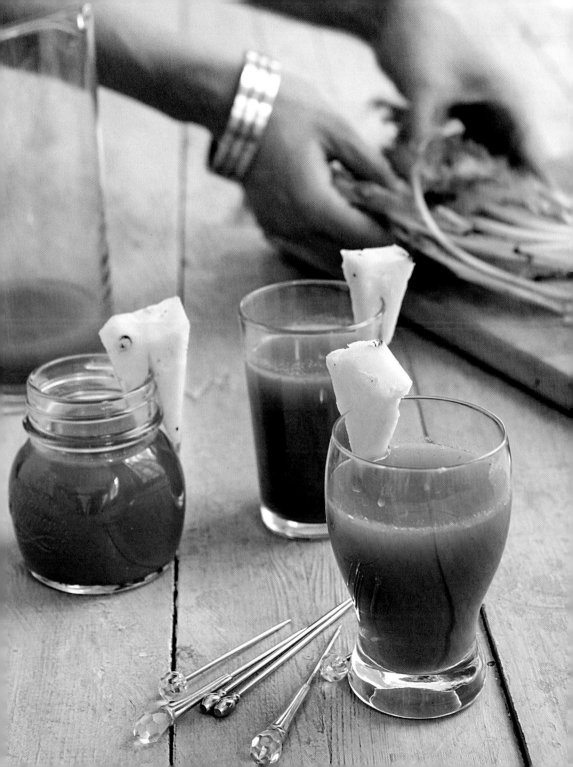

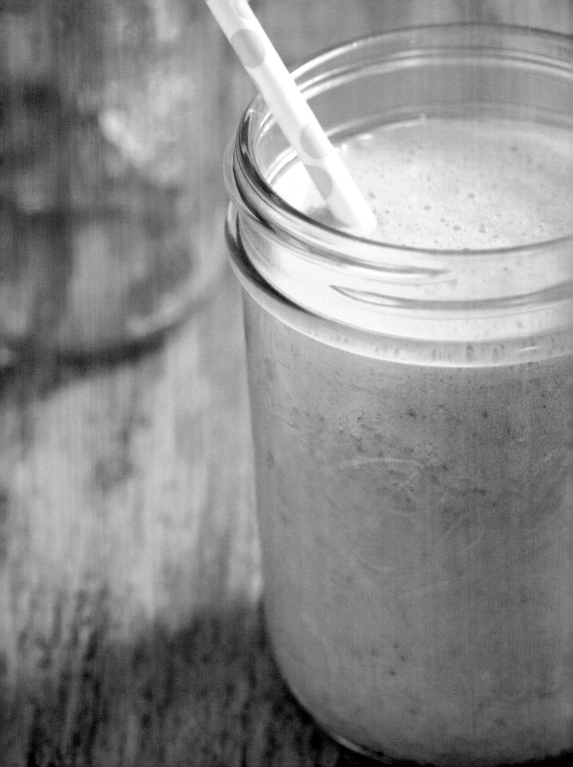

THE ROMAINE LEMONADE

JUICE ❯ ROMAINE LETTUCE, APPLE, LEMON

1 head romaine lettuce

1 Granny Smith apple

½ lemon

Add all ingredients into a juicer and juice.

With fresh romaine, sweet-tart apple, and delicious lemon, this refreshing and rejuvenating combo will have you feeling like a million bucks every A.M.

SERVES 1 ▶ **PER SERVING** 70 CALORIES | 1 G FAT | 4 G PROTEIN | 15 G CARBOHYDRATES | 0 G FIBER | 13 G SUGAR | 550% DV VITAMIN A | 250% DV IRON | 110% DV FOLATE

THE GREEN BANANA-MINT

SMOOTHIE ❯ BABY SPINACH, BANANA, PROTEIN POWDER, MINT, FLAXSEED

1 cup unsweetened almond milk

3 cups baby spinach

1 frozen banana

4 tablespoons (1 scoop) protein powder

3 tablespoons mint

2 tablespoons flaxseeds

1 cup ice

Add ingredients into a blender and blend until smooth.

This smoothie will make you think twice about what green can do for you. Bananas, almond milk, protein powder, and baby spinach?! Don't be shocked if you go bananas for this fortifying green smoothie.

SERVES 4 ▶ **PER SERVING** 140 CALORIES | 4 G FAT | 10 G PROTEIN | 15 G CARBOHYDRATES | 5 G FIBER | 5 G SUGAR | 1,220 MG OMEGA-3 | 15% DV IRON | 20% DV IRON

THE CLEAN GREEN

SMOOTHIE › KALE, BANANA, SPIRULINA, CHIA SEED

1½ cups unsweetened
   coconut milk drink

2 cups kale

1 frozen banana

1 tablespoon spirulina

2 tablespoons chia seeds

1 cup ice

Add ingredients into a
blender and blend until
smooth.

The poster child for this book, the Clean Green is
a delicious and vibrant morning boost to keep you
lean and gorgeous! With kale, filling fiber, and an
immunity boost from spirulina, you're on your way
to reclaiming your health. Go green!

SERVES 3 ▶ **PER SERVING** 120 CALORIES | 5 G FAT | 5 G PROTEIN |
17 G CARBOHYDRATES | 5 G FIBER | 5 G SUGAR | 1,360 MG OMEGA-3 |
520 MG OMEGA-6 | 100% DV VITAMIN A

THE GREEN MONSTER

SMOOTHIE › BABY SPINACH, PEAR, APPLE, GREEN SUPERFOOD

1 cup coconut water

4 cups baby spinach

¾ Bartlett pear, cored

½ Fuji apple

1 teaspoon green
   superfood

1-2 tablespoons lemon
   juice, to taste

1 cup ice

Add ingredients into a
blender and blend until
smooth.

As long as you've got pretty pink nail polish, you'll
still look dainty as ever drinking this MONSTER of a
Clean Green drink! Remember, true beauty starts on
the inside and comes in all shades of green.

SERVES 3 ▶ **PER SERVING** 90 CALORIES | 0 G FAT | 2 G PROTEIN |
20 G CARBOHYDRATES | 5 G FIBER | 10 G SUGAR | 300 MG POTASSIUM |
10% DV CALCIUM | 25% DV IRON

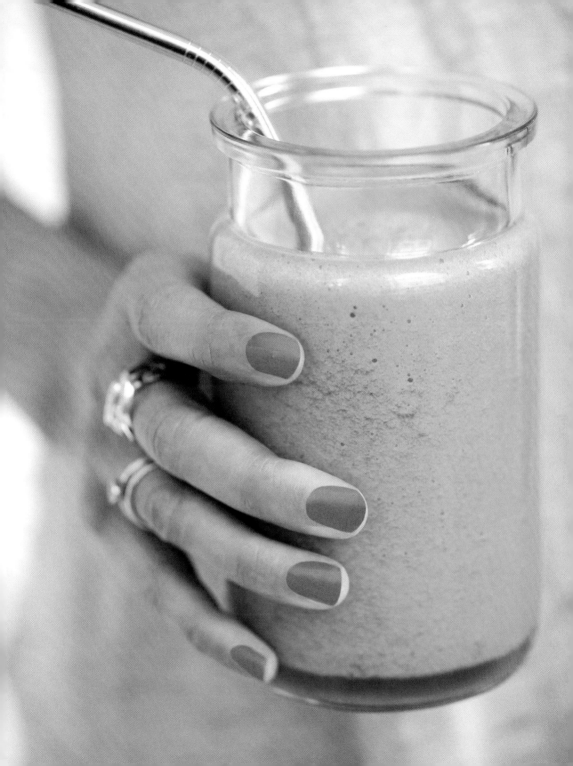

THE KALE BEAUTY ELIXIR

SMOOTHIE › KALE, GREEN SUPERFOOD, BANANA, PEAR

1½ cups unsweetened coconut milk drink

1½ cups kale

2 tablespoons green superfood or spirulina

½ frozen banana

2 Bartlett pears, cored

1 cup ice

Add ingredients into a blender and blend until smooth.

Who doesn't love to feel beautiful and really, really great? That's what the Kale Beauty Elixir will do for you. You can almost feel the nutrients rush into your cells immediately upon sipping this delicious green drink.

SERVES 4 ▶ **PER SERVING** 120 CALORIES | 2.5 G FAT | 3 G PROTEIN | 24 G CARBOHYDRATES | 7 G FIBER | 11 G SUGAR | 20% DV CALCIUM | 35% DV IRON | 10% DV VITAMIN D

THE BLUEBERRY ALMOND

SMOOTHIE › BABY SPINACH, KALE, BLUEBERRY, ALMOND BUTTER, CHIA SEED

2 cups unsweetened almond milk

1 cup baby spinach

1 cup kale

2 cups frozen blueberries

3 tablespoons almond butter

2 tablespoons chia seeds

Add ingredients into a blender and blend until smooth.

Definitely an intermediate-level smoothie, this beautiful blueberry blend is full of real and clean ingredients that will help you glow. Shine on, my love, from the inside out.

SERVES 4 ▶ **PER SERVING** 160 CALORIES | 10 G FAT | 5 G PROTEIN | 16 G CARBOHYDRATES | 6 G FIBER | 7 G SUGAR | 970 MG OMEGA-3 | 40% DV VITAMIN E

98

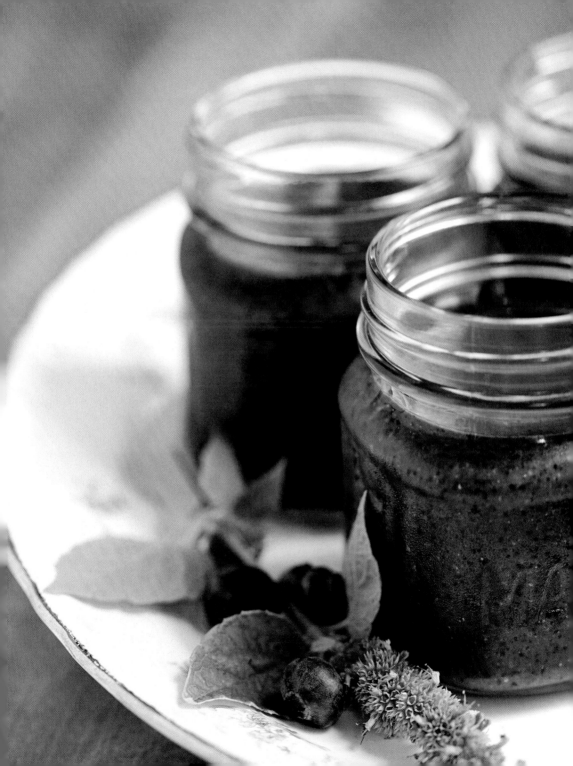

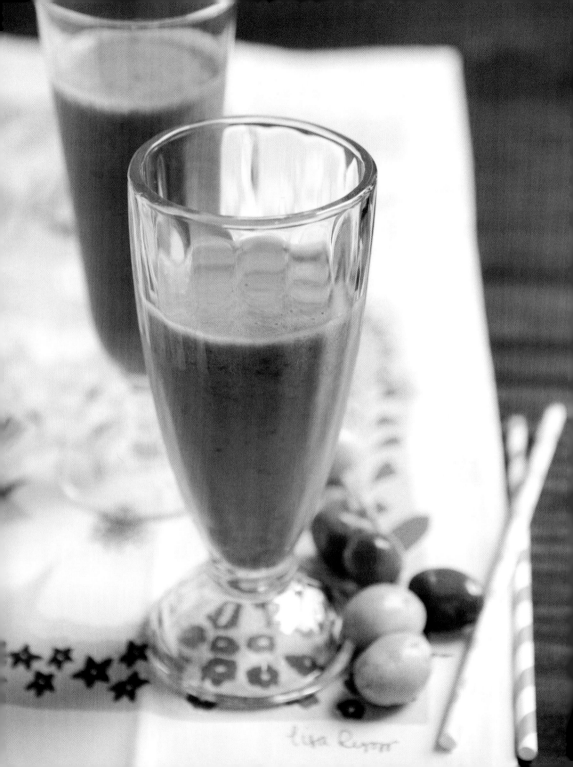

THE DANDELION DATE "SHAKE"

SMOOTHIE ▶ DANDELION, BABY SPINACH, BANANA, DATES

1½ cups unsweetened coconut milk drink

½ cup dandelion greens

2 cups baby spinach

1 frozen banana

3 dried dates, pitted

1 cup ice

Add ingredients into a blender and blend until smooth.

When I was a kid—I must have been six or seven years old—my mom's dear friend Rita used to take us on these incredible trips to Palm Desert, California, where we would sip on date shakes and chill in the sun (while blasting "The Heat Is On," by Glenn Frey, in her fab Cadillac). That was my first experience with the "Date Shake." I'll never forget my first sip: creamy, sweet, delicate, and delicious. With a slightly bitter taste from the dandelion, you will so love this power-punch of greens.

SERVES 2-3 ▶ **PER SERVING** 90 CALORIES | 2.5 G FAT |
1 G PROTEIN | 18 G CARBOHYDRATES | 3 G FIBER | 10 G SUGAR |
270 MG POTASSIUM | 15% DV VITAMIN D

THE GREEN APPLE

SMOOTHIE ❯ KALE, BABY SPINACH, APPLE

1 cup coconut water

1 cup kale

1 cup baby spinach

1½ Fuji apples, cored

⅛ teaspoon cinnamon

⅛ teaspoon nutmeg

1 cup ice

Dash of flaxseed or chia
seeds (optional)

Add ingredients into a
blender and blend until
smooth.

This smoothie has that perfect "apple pie meets
cinnamon and nutmeg" kind of essence. Add in a
touch of flaxseed or chia for an extra fiber boost.

SERVES 4 ▶ **PER SERVING** 70 CALORIES | 0 G FAT | 1 G PROTEIN |
17 G CARBOHYDRATES | 3 G FIBER | 11 G SUGAR | 350 MG POTASSIUM |
50% DV VITAMIN C

THE POPEYE: GREEN MELON
& SPINACH BLEND

SMOOTHIE ❯ BABY SPINACH, BANANA, HONEYDEW MELON

1½ cups unsweetened
coconut milk drink

4 cups baby spinach

1 frozen banana

1½ cups honeydew melon,
cubed

1 cup ice (optional)

Add ingredients into a
blender and blend until
smooth.

If you love spinach and all things sweet and green,
you will love this delicious and refreshing beverage.
Go, Popeye! He was no joke.

SERVES 4 ▶ **PER SERVING** 80 CALORIES | 2 G FAT | 1 G PROTEIN |
16 G CARBOHYDRATES | 3 G FIBER | 9 G SUGAR | 10% DV VITAMIN D

Measuring Greens

When you're in a hurry, or you become a self-proclaimed pro at blending and juicing, you're not really going to care much for precision anymore. Here are a few tips to help measure greens in a flash.

Green Herbs	Spinach	Kale
5 basil or mint leaves = approximately 1 tablespoon	Wash thoroughly, pat dry, and rough chop before measuring; 1 handful of chopped spinach = approximately 1 cup	Remove woody stems from kale and rough chop before measuring; 1 handful of chopped kale = approximately 1 cup
Romaine/Red Leaf Romaine	**Dandelion/ Mizuna**	**Baby Spinach/ Arugula**
Wash thoroughly, pat dry, and rough chop before measuring; 1 handful of chopped romaine = approximately 1 cup	Wash thoroughly, pat dry, remove ends and stems, and rough chop before measuring; 1 handful of chopped dandelion/mizuna = approximately 1 cup	1 handful of baby spinach or arugula = approximately 1 cup

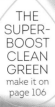

THE
SUPER-
BOOST
CLEAN
GREEN
make it on
page 106

6

> *"Super greens make for a superhuman kind of day."* —CK

Super Energy-Boosting Juices & Smoothies

FOR AN IMMEDIATE jolt to fight off that midday slump, these naturally derived, unprocessed Clean Green drinks will have you feeling like a champion. Let all those organic nutrients flow in and all of your deep breaths flow out. Good, clean energy is here to fuel your day.

THE SUPER-BOOST CLEAN GREEN

SMOOTHIE ❯ KALE, BABY SPINACH, GREEN SUPERFOOD, BANANA, GINGER, ALMOND BUTTER

1½ cups unsweetened almond milk

1 cup kale

2 cups baby spinach

1 teaspoon green super-food or spirulina

1½ frozen bananas

3 teaspoons fresh ginger

2 tablespoons almond butter

1 cup ice

Add ingredients into a blender and blend until smooth.

This recipe was created for the smoothie-lover who's got no fear of super-healthy freshness. With ginger, spinach, green superfood, spirulina, almond butter, and everything but the kitchen sink, you'll love this combo pre- or post-workout.

SERVES 4 ▶ **PER SERVING** 120 CALORIES | 6 G FAT | 4 G PROTEIN | 16 G CARBOHYDRATES | 4 G FIBER | 6 G SUGAR | 15% DV CALCIUM | 10% DV IRON | 30% DV VITAMIN E

THE EVERYTHING!

JUICE ❯ CARROT, BABY SPINACH, PINEAPPLE, CUCUMBER

3 organic carrots, scrubbed

5 cups baby spinach

1 cup fresh pineapple

1 large cucumber

⅛ teaspoon cinnamon

Add all ingredients into a juicer and juice. Then whisk in the cinnamon to combine.

After a few weeks of Clean Green, I know you'll want to try to juice absolutely everything, from the veggies in Grandma's backyard to the locally grown mint at the farmer's market. I've already thrown just about everything into this next juice. Why the heck not? Live clean, green, and happily.

SERVES 2 ▶ **PER SERVING** 80 CALORIES | 0.5 G FAT | 3 G PROTEIN | 19 G CARBOHYDRATES | 0 G FIBER | 14 G SUGAR | 570 MG POTASSIUM | 350% DV VITAMIN A | 100% DV VITAMIN C

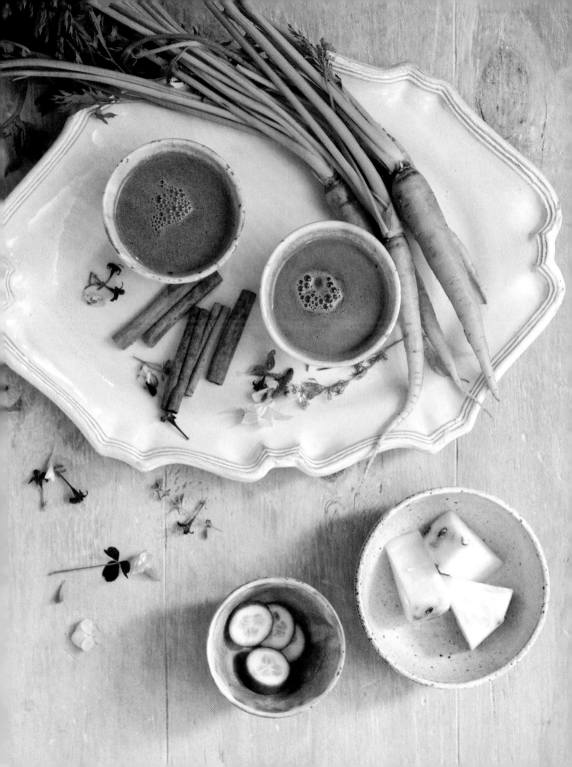

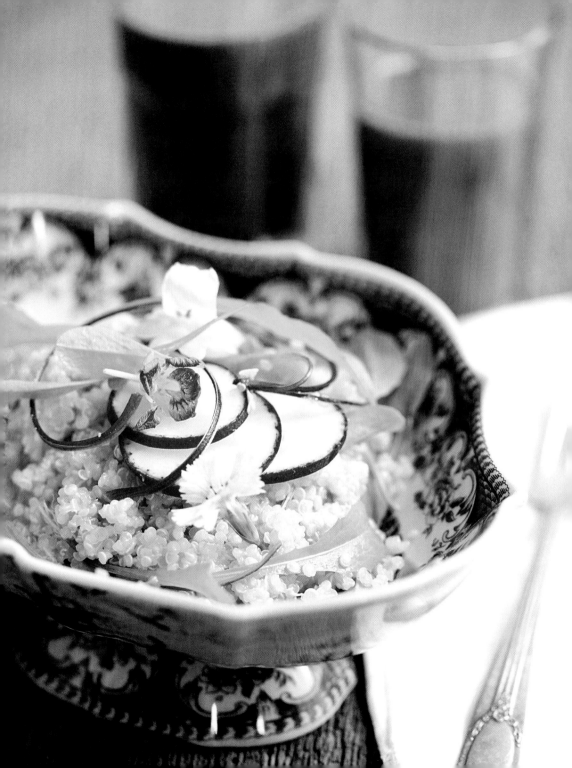

THE MANGO-KALE KICK

JUICE › BABY SPINACH, KALE, MANGO

3 cups baby spinach

1 cup kale

½ ripe mango, pitted, sliced

1 cup coconut water

Add the spinach, kale, and ripe mango. Juice, then add the coconut water, whisking well to combine.

Mango-kale madness! I like to call this recipe the Mango-Kale Kick, because we all need a kick in the pants during a midday slump, right? Add some zing to that Clean Green lifestyle.

SERVES 1 ▶ **PER SERVING** 170 CALORIES | 1.5 G FAT | 6 G PROTEIN | 38 G CARBOHYDRATES | 0 G FIBER | 30 G SUGAR | 1,080 MG POTASSIUM | 20% DV CALCIUM | 25% DV FOLATE

THE CARROT DANDELION

JUICE › CARROT, BABY SPINACH, DANDELION, GINGER, APPLE

½ pound organic carrots, scrubbed

2 cups baby spinach

¾ cup dandelion greens

1 tablespoon fresh ginger

½ Fuji apple

Add all ingredients into a juicer and juice.

The bitterness of dandelion, balanced by the organic sweetness of carrots, makes this clean drink the hottest way to detox after a Friday night out with the girls. With fresh ginger and yummy greens, say good-bye to that headache the natural way.

SERVES 1 ▶ **PER SERVING** 120 CALORIES | 1 G FAT | 4 G PROTEIN | 28 G CARBOHYDRATES | 0 G FIBER | 19 G SUGAR | 1,000 MG POTASSIUM | 880% DV VITAMIN A | 20% DV CALCIUM

THE SPICY-GINGER
PINEAPPLE GREEN

JUICE › PINEAPPLE, BABY SPINACH, GINGER, CUCUMBER

¾ cup fresh pineapple

3 cups baby spinach

1 tablespoon fresh ginger

1 medium cucumber

Add all ingredients into a juicer and juice. Then whisk in cinnamon.

Such a beautiful marriage. You know when two things come together, and it's just magic? That's ginger and pineapple. Enjoy this delicious and satisfying cleansing juice.

SERVES 1-2 › **PER SERVING** 90 CALORIES | 0.5 G FAT | 3 G PROTEIN | 19 G CARBOHYDRATES | 0 G FIBER | 15 G SUGAR | 130% DV VITAMIN C | 10% DV CALCIUM | 15% DV IRON

THE HAWAIIAN-GREEN
PINEAPPLE PUNCH

SMOOTHIE › BABY SPINACH, BANANA, PINEAPPLE, BEE POLLEN

1½ cups unsweetened coconut milk drink

2 cups baby spinach

1 frozen banana

1 cup fresh pineapple

1 teaspoon spirulina

1 teaspoon bee pollen

1 cup ice

Add ingredients into a blender and blend until smooth.

If you're into something slightly exotic, this smoothie will whisk you away to the islands! Fresh pineapple, coconut milk drink, banana, and spirulina—sounds like a healthy, fresh, and "green" version of a Lava Flow cocktail! Okole maluna!

SERVES 4 › **PER SERVING** 70 CALORIES | 2 G FAT | 1 G PROTEIN | 15 G CARBOHYDRATES | 2 G FIBER | 8 G SUGAR | 10% DV VITAMIN D

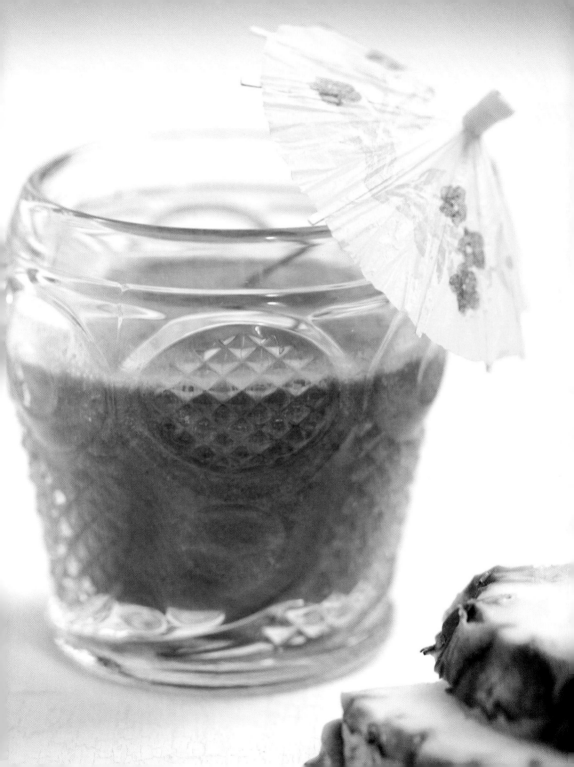

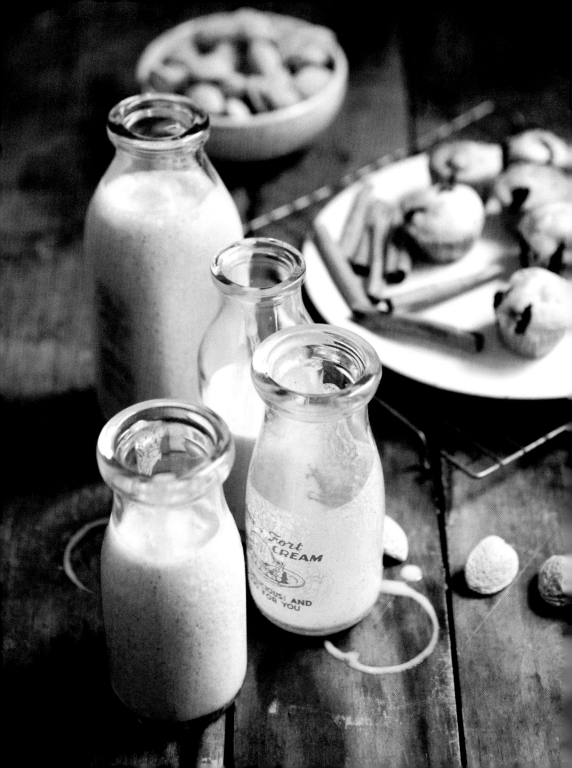

THE CINNAMON-ALMOND HORCHATA

SMOOTHIE > BANANA, MACA, ALMOND BUTTER

1 cup unsweetened almond milk

1 frozen banana

1 teaspoon cinnamon

1 tablespoon maca powder

2 tablespoons almond butter

1 cup ice

Add ingredients into a blender and blend until smooth.

This absolutely delicious recipe was developed for my crew with our beloved California in mind. With cinnamon, maca root, and almond butter, this creamy and satisfying smoothie will give you happy energy. All smiles.

SERVES 2 ▶ **PER SERVING** 200 CALORIES | 10 G FAT | 6 G PROTEIN | 24 G CARBOHYDRATES | 6 G FIBER | 10 G SUGAR | 20% DV CALCIUM | 45% DV VITAMIN E

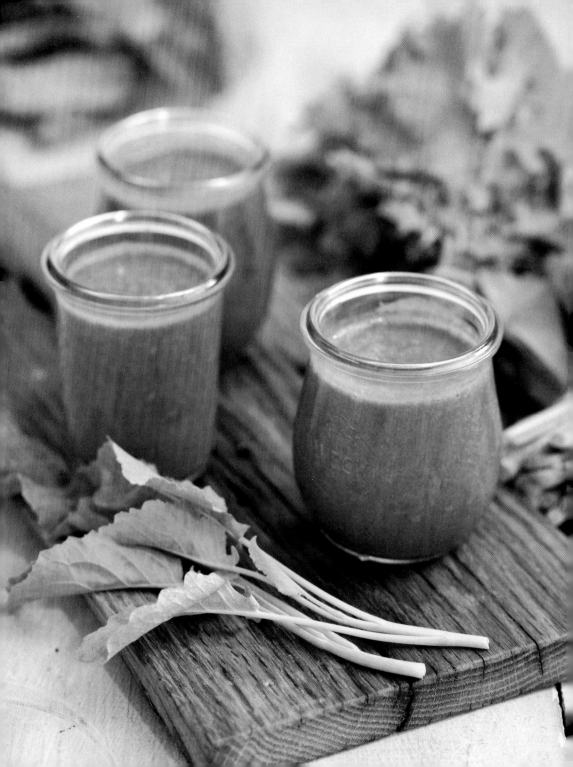

THE AÇAI SUPER BERRY
SMOOTHIE > AÇAI, BABY SPINACH, GREEN SUPERFOOD

2 100-gram açai frozen
  berry packs (by
  Sambazon)
2 cups baby spinach
1 frozen banana
1¼ cups coconut water
1 tablespoon spirulina
1 tablespoon green
  superfood

Add ingredients into a
blender and blend until
smooth.

With all the hype, the açai berry certainly is packed with antioxidants and will improve your overall health. Be good to super-you. Look for this berry in the freezer section at your local health food store.

SERVES 3 ▶ **PER SERVING** 130 CALORIES | 4 G FAT | 4 G PROTEIN | 21 G CARBOHYDRATES | 5 G FIBER | 10 G SUGAR | 440 MG POTASSIUM | 10% DV CALCIUM | 30% DV IRON

THE SUPER GREEN MANGO
SMOOTHIE > KALE, MANGO, SPIRULINA

2½ cups unsweetened
   almond milk
1½ cups kale
3 cups frozen mango
1 tablespoon spirulina

Add ingredients into a
blender and blend until
smooth.

If you love brunch on the weekends with friends, I suggest blending up this remedy for all of your guests! With creamy mango, nutrient-bursting kale, and your new favorite—spirulina—your friends are gonna heart you even more.

SERVES 4 ▶ **PER SERVING** 130 CALORIES | 2.5 G FAT | 4 G PROTEIN | 28 G CARBOHYDRATES | 4 G FIBER | 21 G SUGAR | 110% DV VITAMIN C | 15% DV CALCIUM | 35% DV VITAMIN E

THE PEANUT BUTTER BOOSTER

SMOOTHIE ▷ BANANA, PINEAPPLE, PEANUT BUTTER, MACA

1 cup unsweetened almond milk

1 frozen banana

½ cup pineapple

2 tablespoons natural peanut butter

2 tablespoons maca root powder

1 cup ice

Add ingredients into a blender and blend until smooth.

If you don't love peanut butter, don't look! For everyone else, this absolutely delicious treat will have you going nuts over its incredible flavor, not to mention the natural energy boost you'll get from the maca root powder. Think organic boosters, not chemical-laden energy drinks. Be good to your body and mind.

SERVES 2 ▶ **PER SERVING** 250 CALORIES | 10 G FAT | 8 G PROTEIN | 36 G CARBOHYDRATES | 7 G FIBER | 16 G SUGAR | 10% DV IRON | 10% DV VITAMIN D | 25% DV VITAMIN E

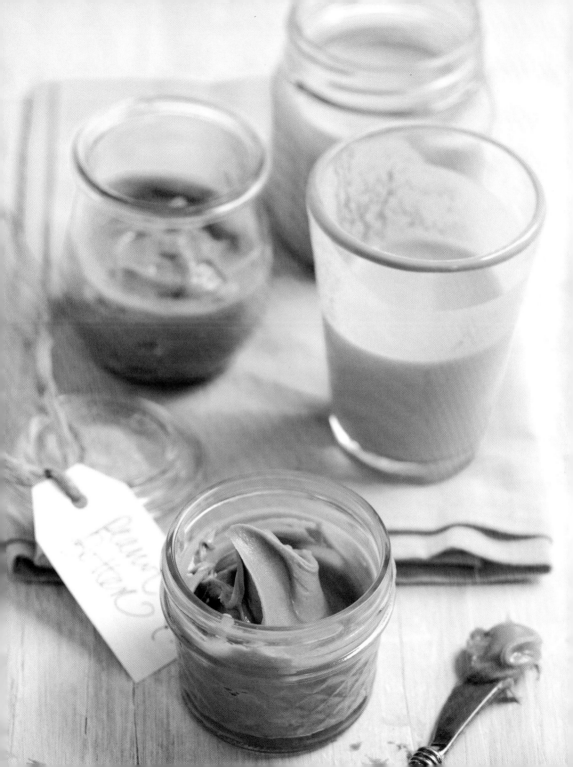

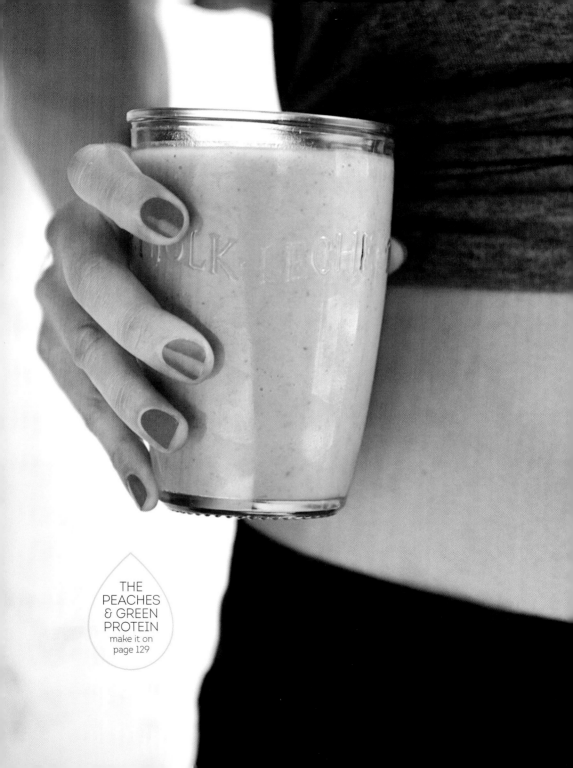

THE
PEACHES
& GREEN
PROTEIN
make it on
page 129

"Healing is a matter of time, but it is sometimes also a matter of opportunity." –HIPPOCRATES

7

Post-Work-out Lean-Protein Smoothies

WHEN I BEGAN writing for men's nutrition-and-wellness publications, I wasn't too keen on their obsession with protein powders. Yet, as I began to research and experience the wonders of ingredients like natural hemp protein, rice protein, and pea protein, I soon became a fan. Within weeks of testing these post-workout smoothies, my body leaned up; and I had just as much muscle tone as I did when I was running half marathons.

THE GREEN VANILLA ALMOND
(TASTES LIKE A VANILLA SHAKE—OMG!)
SMOOTHIE › BABY SPINACH, BANANA, ALMOND BUTTER, PROTEIN POWDER

1 **cup unsweetened coconut water**

2 **cups baby spinach**

1 **frozen banana**

2 **tablespoons almond butter**

2 **teaspoons organic vanilla extract**

4 **tablespoons (1 scoop) protein powder**

1 **cup ice**

Add ingredients into a blender and blend until smooth.

While developing and testing this recipe with my team, we all went a little crazy for it. Everyone kept going back for seconds, since it tastes just like a vanilla milkshake! But you're actually slurping on nutrient-rich spinach, almond butter, and coconut water. Get it, gorgeous. Beauty starts from the inside; it's just a bonus that it can taste this good.

SERVES 2 ▶ **PER SERVING** 180 CALORIES | 6 G FAT | 11 G PROTEIN | 17 G CARBOHYDRATES | 3 G FIBER | 8 G SUGAR | 380 MG POTASSIUM | 20% DV IRON | 15% DV VITAMIN E

THE BLUEBERRY PROTEIN POWER "SHAKE"
SMOOTHIE › BANANA, BLUEBERRY, PROTEIN POWDER

2 **cups unsweetened almond milk**

1 **frozen banana**

2 **cups frozen blueberries**

4 **tablespoons (1 scoop) protein powder**

1 **cup ice**

Add ingredients into a blender and blend until smooth.

Need a little lean "boost" for that developing six-pack? Try this Blueberry Protein Power "Shake" (I prefer mine with pea protein). It will have you doing lean-protein backflips in no time.

SERVES 2-4 ▶ **PER SERVING** 140 CALORIES | 3 G FAT | 9 G PROTEIN | 18 G CARBOHYDRATES | 4 G FIBER | 10 G SUGAR | 15% DV CALCIUM | 15% DV VITAMIN D | 35% DV VITAMIN E

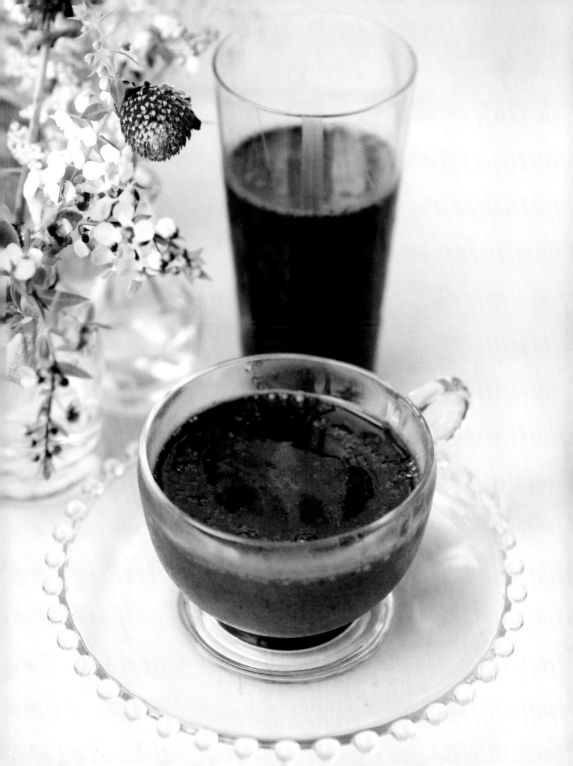

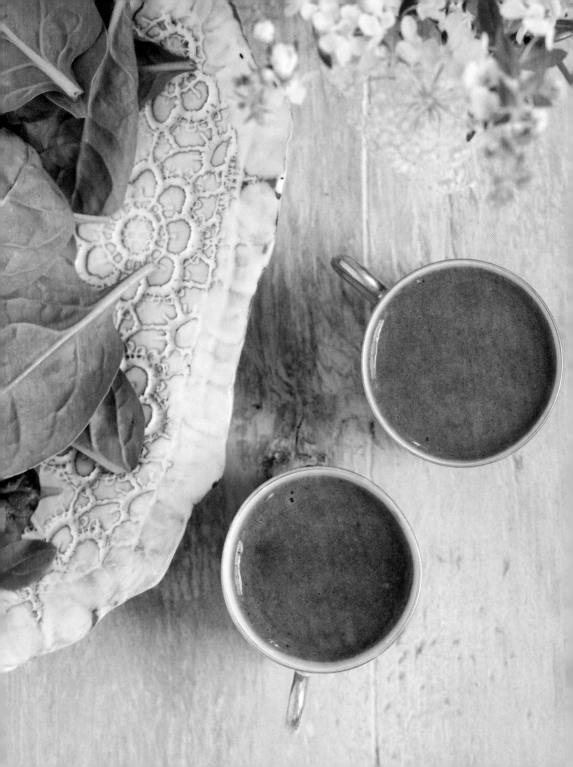

THE GREEN MANGO BOOSTER

SMOOTHIE ❯ BABY SPINACH, MANGO, BANANA, BEE POLLEN, SPIRULINA

1¼ cups unsweetened almond milk

2 cups baby spinach

1 cup frozen mango

1 frozen banana

1 teaspoon bee pollen

2 teaspoons spirulina

4 tablespoons (1 scoop) protein powder

Add ingredients into a blender and blend until smooth.

If you love the luscious combo of banana and mango, you'll love this naturally boosting smoothie. With bee pollen and spirulina, you can't go wrong sipping this green treat!

SERVES 3 ▶ **PER SERVING** 160 CALORIES | 1.5 G FAT |
11 G PROTEIN | 24 G CARBOHYDRATES | 4 G FIBER | 14 G SUGAR |
20% DV IRON | 20% DV VITAMIN E

THE LEAN PUMPKIN "SHAKE"

SMOOTHIE › PUMPKIN PUREE, BANANA, PEAR, PROTEIN POWDER

1½ cups unsweetened almond milk

¾ cup organic pumpkin puree

1 frozen banana

½ Bartlett pear, cored

¼ teaspoon pumpkin spice

4 tablespoons (1 scoop) protein powder

½ cup ice

Add ingredients into a blender and blend until smooth.

One of my most popular smoothies to date, starring delicious, vitamin-A-loaded pumpkin puree. You are hooking yourself up here, hon. Whip up an extra glass for your man or a girlfriend at work, and share the satiety and nutrition together.

SERVES 2 ▶ **PER SERVING** 140 CALORIES | 2 G FAT | 10 G PROTEIN | 19 G CARBOHYDRATES | 5 G FIBER | 10 G SUGAR | 160% DV VITAMIN A | 15% DV CALCIUM | 15% DV IRON

THE BANANA MUSCLE

SMOOTHIE › BABY SPINACH, BANANA, ALMOND BUTTER, PROTEIN POWDER

1 cup unsweetened almond milk

1 cup baby spinach

1½ frozen bananas

2 tablespoons almond butter

4 tablespoons (1 scoop) protein powder

1 cup ice

Add ingredients into a blender and blend until smooth.

My friend Tina totally makes fun of me for my outlandish recipe titles. But, hey, they work. You're going to remember banana, lean muscle, and sexy body, right? Think when you drink.

SERVES 4 ▶ **PER SERVING** 270 CALORIES | 11 G FAT | 16 G PROTEIN | 26 G CARBOHYDRATES | 5 G FIBER | 12 G SUGAR | 530 MG POTASSIUM | 25% DV IRON | 45% DV VITAMIN E

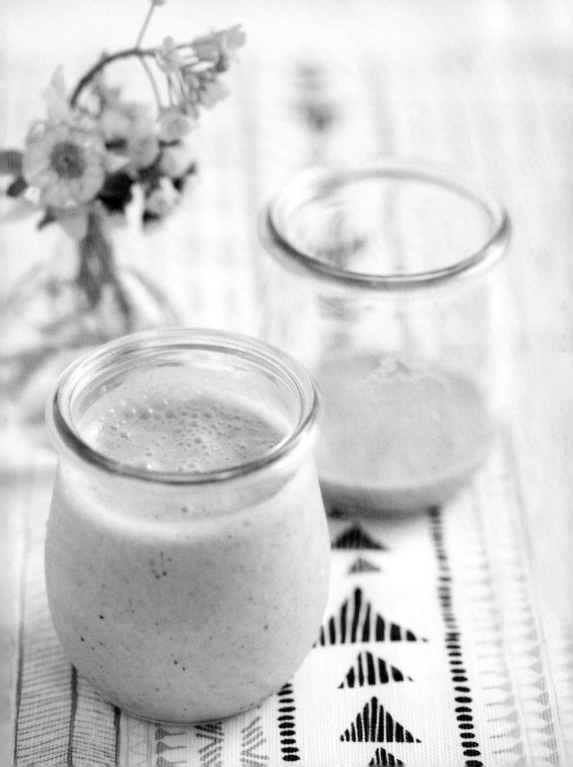

THE CHOCOLATE PEANUT BUTTER MONSTER

SMOOTHIE › BABY SPINACH, BANANA, PEAR, PEANUT BUTTER, CHOCOLATE

1 cup unsweetened almond milk

2 cups baby spinach

1 frozen banana

½ Bartlett pear, cored

2 tablespoons natural peanut butter

2 tablespoons unsweetened cocoa powder

1 cup ice

Add ingredients into a blender and blend until smooth.

This is truly like heaven in a glass. Every friend who tested this recipe had to send a text: "Oh, my goodness, it tastes like a chocolate peanut butter cup!" Happy tummies and happy friends. That's what I strive for. Can't wait to receive your text, tweet, or post. Enjoy!

SERVES 3 ▶ **PER SERVING** 150 CALORIES | 7 G FAT | 4 G PROTEIN | 20 G CARBOHYDRATES | 5 G FIBER | 8 G SUGAR | 290 MG POTASSIUM | 15% DV VITAMIN E

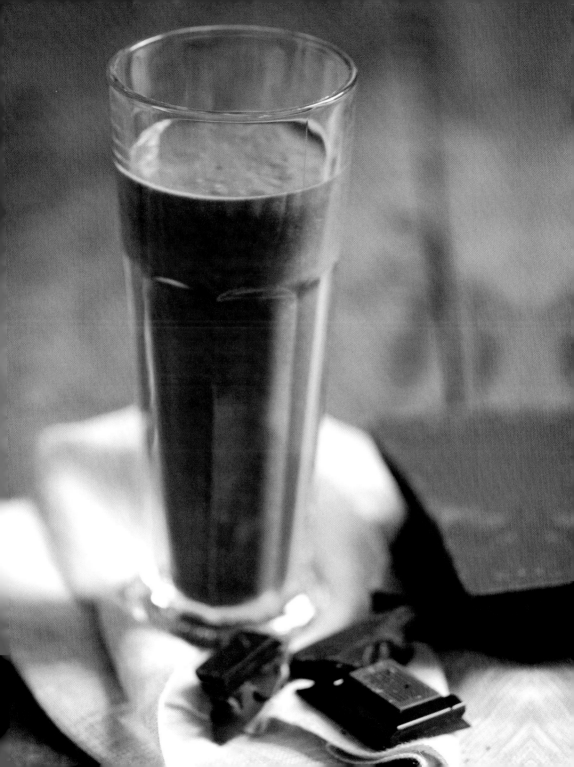

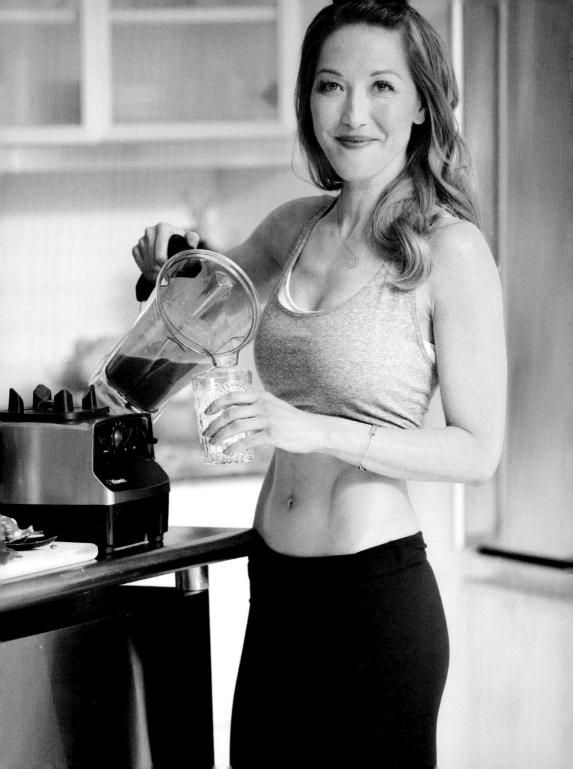

THE PEACHES AND GREEN PROTEIN

SMOOTHIE › BABY SPINACH, GREEN SUPERFOOD, PEACH, PROTEIN POWDER

1¾ cups unsweetened almond milk

2 cups baby spinach

½ cup kale

1 tablespoon green superfood

½ frozen banana

2 cups frozen peaches

1 teaspoon spirulina

4 tablespoons (1 scoop) protein powder

Add ingredients into a blender and blend until smooth.

If you haven't experienced the wonders of pea protein yet, I suggest you give it a little test. How can you go wrong with 9 grams of protein per serving and 30 percent of your daily recommended iron? You're all set, sister. Keep working out and living green and lean!

SERVES 4 ▶ **PER SERVING** 120 CALORIES | 1.5 G FAT | 9 G PROTEIN | 16 G CARBOHYDRATES | 4 G FIBER | 8 G SUGAR | 130% DV VITAMIN C | 30% DV IRON

THE SUPERFOOD
CHOCOLATE BOOSTER

SMOOTHIE › BABY SPINACH, GREEN SUPERFOOD, SPIRULINA, BANANA,
CHOCOLATE, PROTEIN POWDER

1¼ cups unsweetened
almond milk

1 cup baby spinach

1 tablespoon green
superfood

1 tablespoon spirulina

1 frozen banana

2 tablespoons unsweet-
ened cocoa powder

4 tablespoons (1 scoop)
protein powder

1 teaspoon bee pollen
(optional)

1 teaspoon probiotics
powder (optional)

1 cup ice

Add ingredients into a
blender and blend until
smooth.

If you want a super-chocolatey boost of protein
after your workout, then this is your cocoa-lover's
choice. With everything from green superfood and
spirulina to spinach and cocoa powder, plus bee
pollen and probiotics, you're destined to be
Superwoman after this lean drink.

SERVES 2 ▶ **PER SERVING** 200 CALORIES | 3.5 G FAT |
18 G PROTEIN | 25 G CARBOHYDRATES | 7 G FIBER | 8 G SUGAR |
570 MG POTASSIUM | 25% DV CALCIUM | 60% DV IRON | 30% DV VITAMIN E

Green Baking

SAVE THE EXCESS PULP FROM YOUR JUICER and throw it into muffins, breads, and pancakes, or even toss some into your soups and stir-fries. Don't let all of that nutrient-dense pulp go to waste! And then how about composting what remains?

THE SUPER HEMP

SMOOTHIE › BABY SPINACH, GREEN SUPERFOOD, BANANA, BLUEBERRY, HEMP PROTEIN POWDER

1 cup coconut almond milk

1 cup baby spinach

1 tablespoon green superfood

½ frozen banana

2 cups frozen blueberries

2 tablespoons hemp protein powder

1 tablespoon spirulina

1 teaspoon hempseed oil (optional)

Add ingredients into a blender and blend until smooth.

This sexy hemp smoothie is a must-try. You will love the nutty and earthy taste of hemp! Mmm, who doesn't? Hemp is definitely a feel-good, good-for-you super-booster, I highly recommend adding hemp to your hot and cold cereals, baked goods, and breakfast scrambles.

SERVES 2 ▶ **PER SERVING** 180 CALORIES | 3.5 G FAT | 9 G PROTEIN | 33 G CARBOHYDRATES | 11 G FIBER | 16 G SUGAR | 250 MG OMEGA-3 | 35% DV CALCIUM | 50% DV IRON | 10% DV VITAMIN D

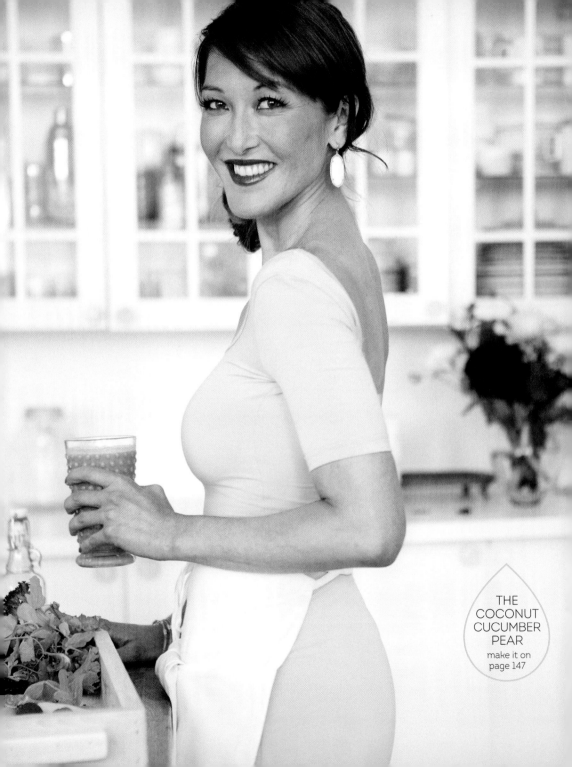

THE
COCONUT
CUCUMBER
PEAR

make it on
page 147

Skin–Cleansing Juices & Smoothies

8

HYDRATING, ANTI–INFLAMMATORY, skin-calming drinks. Sounds soothing and fabulous, right? For years I fought with irritated, sensitive, acne-prone skin. It was a nightmare, until I discovered the benefits of Clean Green drinks. You're probably asking yourself, "How can Clean Green smoothies and juices help the appearance of my skin?"

Simple: Antioxidant and enzyme consumption helps fight free radicals, which are unstable atoms that may lead to conditions worse than wrinkles. Thus, you want to fight them in any way you can. It is all about prevention.

Start drinking cleaner and greener and you may notice real improvements in your skin. For an even greater beauty boost, drink plenty of water and wear sunscreen every day! Take good care of yourself, gorgeous.

THE CARROT CAKE
JUICE › BABY SPINACH, CARROT, APPLE

4 cups baby spinach

1 pound bag of organic carrots, scrubbed

½ Fuji apple

¼ teaspoon ground cinnamon

¼ teaspoon pumpkin spice

Juice the spinach, carrots, and apple into a glass. Add cinnamon and pumpkin spice; whisk well to combine.

If you love the natural sweetness of carrots and the warmth of fragrant pumpkin spice, give this juice a squeeze. It tastes like a delicious bite of your favorite carrot cake!

SERVES 2 (SMALL GLASSES) ▶ **PER SERVING** 90 CALORIES 0.5 G FAT ⋮ 3 G PROTEIN ⋮ 21 G CARBOHYDRATES ⋮ 0 G FIBER ⋮ 15 G SUGAR ⋮ 770 MG POTASSIUM ⋮ 790% DV VITAMIN A ⋮ 10% DV FOLATE

Alkaline Balance

ALKALIZING REFERS TO MAINTAINING the body's ideal pH balance, which is, according to American Dietetic Association spokeswoman Marjorie Nolan, R.D.,"between 7.35 and 7.45, no matter how we eat." You can get there with the natural help of lemons, which contain citric acid that can keep your body properly balanced. According to Phyllis A. Balch, C.N.C., in *Prescription for Dietary Wellness*, "Lemon juice has antibacterial properties and can be used to cleanse the system, purify the blood..., and balance the pH (the level of acidity) in the colon. Diluted with quality water, it can be used as a cleansing enema to detoxify the system."

THE KALE GLOW

JUICE › KALE, BABY SPINACH, PEAR, CUCUMBER

3 cups kale

1 cup baby spinach

½ Bosc pear, cored

1 cucumber

¼ lemon

Add all ingredients into a juicer and juice.

We all want to shine sometimes, right? Get your glow on with natural ingredients like kale, cucumber, and purifying lemon! #Glow #CleanGreen

SERVES 1 ▶ **PER SERVING** 150 CALORIES | 2.5 G FAT |
11 G PROTEIN | 28 G CARBOHYDRATES | 0 G FIBER | 12 G SUGAR |
360 MG OMEGA-3 | 1,362 MG POTASSIUM | 430% DV VITAMIN C

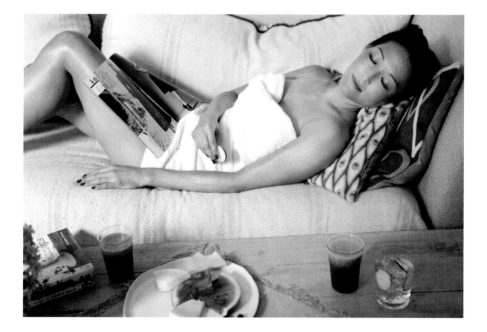

THE CUCUMBER-MINT-COCONUT CLEANSER

JUICE ▷ CUCUMBER, BABY SPINACH, APPLE, MINT

1 medium cucumber

3 cups baby spinach

¼ Fuji apple

5 tablespoons fresh mint

1 cup coconut water

Juice cucumber, spinach, apple, and mint into a glass. Add the coconut water and whisk well to combine.

Doesn't it feel absolutely wonderful when you can make it to the spa to detox and re-energize over the weekend? Why not invite some of your besties over for a spa day and relax with this delicious, skin-brightening treat?

SERVES 2 ▶ **PER SERVING** 45 CALORIES | 0 G FAT | 1 G PROTEIN | 9 G CARBOHYDRATES | 0 G FIBER | 7 G SUGAR | 410 MG POTASSIUM | 30% DV VITAMIN A | 8% DV IRON

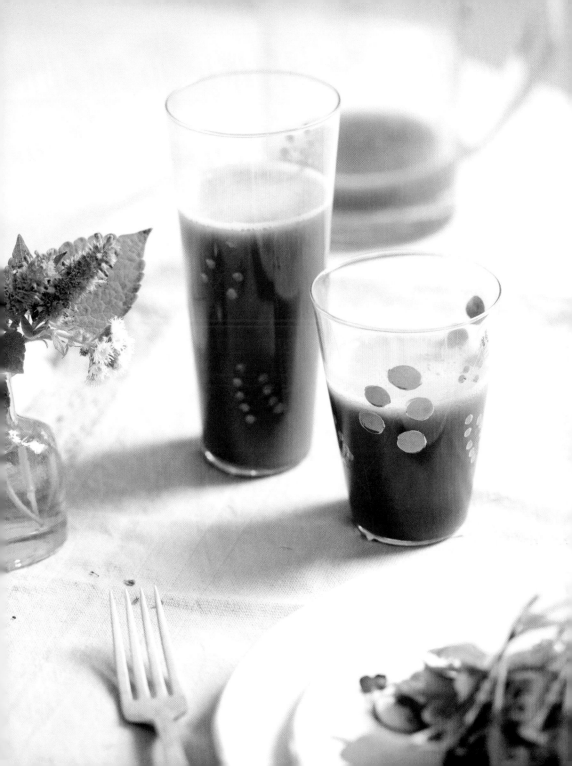

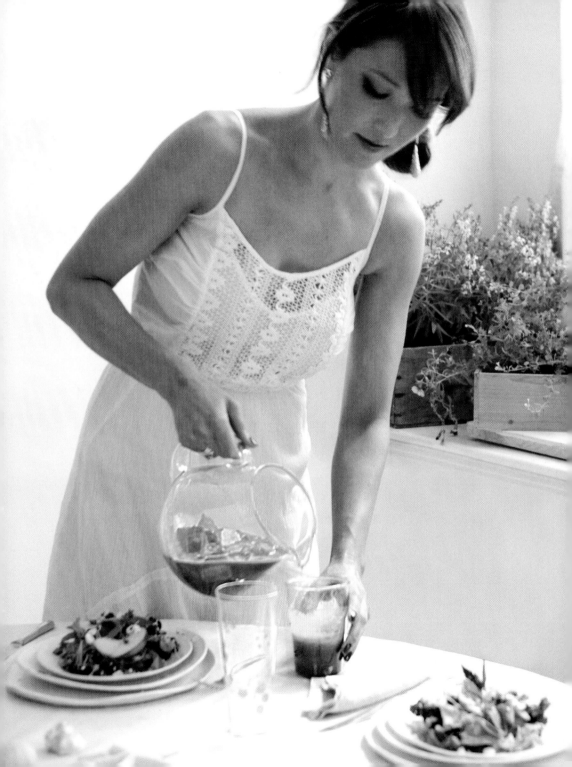

THE GINGER PEACH

JUICE > KALE, BABY SPINACH, GINGER, PEACH

2 cups kale

5 cups baby spinach

1 teaspoon fresh ginger

¾ peach, pitted

¼ cup coconut water

Juice kale, spinach, ginger, and sliced peach into a glass. Add the coconut water and whisk well to combine.

This delicious and fresh combination of peaches, ginger, kale, and coconut water will have you feeling and looking hydrated and fresh, naturally. Who needs beauty serums and topical tonics, when you can glow from within?

SERVES 2 ▶ **PER SERVING** 120 CALORIES | 1.5 G FAT | 9 G PROTEIN | 22 G CARBOHYDRATES | 0 G FIBER | 11 G SUGAR | 240 MG OMEGA-3 | 310% DV VITAMIN C | 30% DV CALCIUM

THE SWEET POTATO PEACH

SMOOTHIE > BANANA, SWEET POTATO PUREE, PEACH, PROTEIN POWDER

2½ cups unsweetened almond milk

½ frozen banana

¾ cup sweet potato puree, or steamed sweet potatoes

3 cups frozen, organic peaches

¼ teaspoon pumpkin spice

¼ teaspoon nutmeg

¼ teaspoon cinnamon

4 tablespoons (1 scoop) protein powder (optional)

Add ingredients into a blender and blend until smooth.

Sweet potato, brimming with vitamin A and fiber, can also help boost your immune system as well as your mood! Enjoy, and feel good about your new Clean Green life!

SERVES 4 ▶ **PER SERVING** 120 CALORIES | 2 G FAT | 2 G PROTEIN | 25 G CARBOHYDRATES | 3 G FIBER | 13 G SUGAR | 460 MG POTASSIUM | 180% DV VITAMIN C | 15% DV VITAMIN D

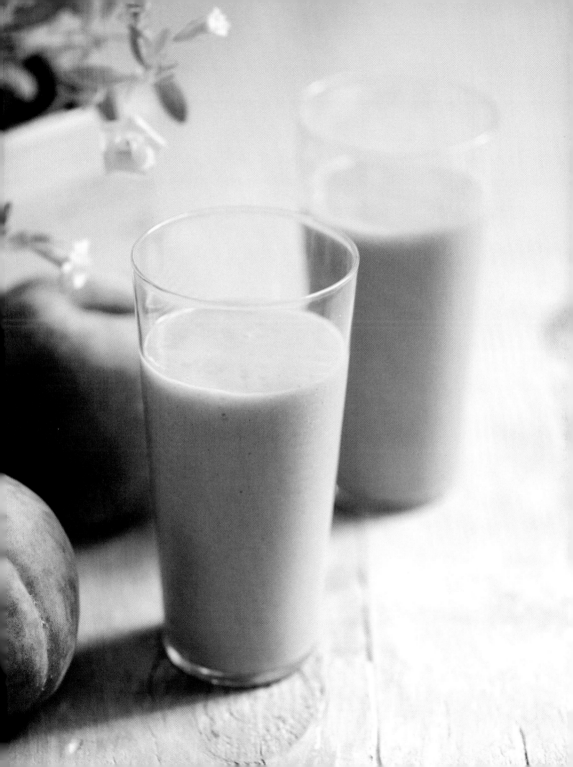

THE GREEN PUMPKIN

SMOOTHIE ❯ BABY SPINACH, PEAR, BANANA, PUMPKIN PUREE, PROTEIN POWDER

1½ cups unsweetened almond milk

2 cups baby spinach

1 Bartlett pear, cored

½ frozen banana

¾ cup pumpkin puree

2 tablespoons protein powder (optional)

Add ingredients into a blender and blend until smooth.

Pumpkin, with its amazing supple-skin benefits, can also be great on the skin's exterior. So sip on this delicious green drink while smoothing on your pumpkin enzyme mask for double bennies.

SERVES 3 ▶ **PER SERVING** 100 CALORIES : 2 G FAT : 2 G PROTEIN : 21 G CARBOHYDRATES : 6 G FIBER : 10 G SUGAR : 170% DV VITAMIN A : 15% DV CALCIUM : 25% DV VITAMIN E

THE CREAMY PUMPKIN PIE

SMOOTHIE ❯ BANANA, PEAR, PUMPKIN PUREE, GINGER

1½ cups unsweetened almond milk

2 frozen bananas

1 Bartlett pear, cored

½ cup pumpkin puree

1 tablespoon grated ginger

¼ teaspoon pumpkin spice

1 cup ice

Add ingredients into a blender and blend until smooth.

Pumpkin pie in a glass? Yum! With vitamins A, B3, B5, B6, and C; potassium; and fiber, how can you say no to all of these bennies with each sip? Drink to your health and get even more radiant!

SERVES 4 ▶ **PER SERVING** 110 CALORIES : 1.5 G FAT : 2 G PROTEIN : 23 G CARBOHYDRATES : 5 G FIBER : 13 G SUGAR : 80% DV VITAMIN A : 10% DV VITAMIN D : 20% DV VITAMIN E

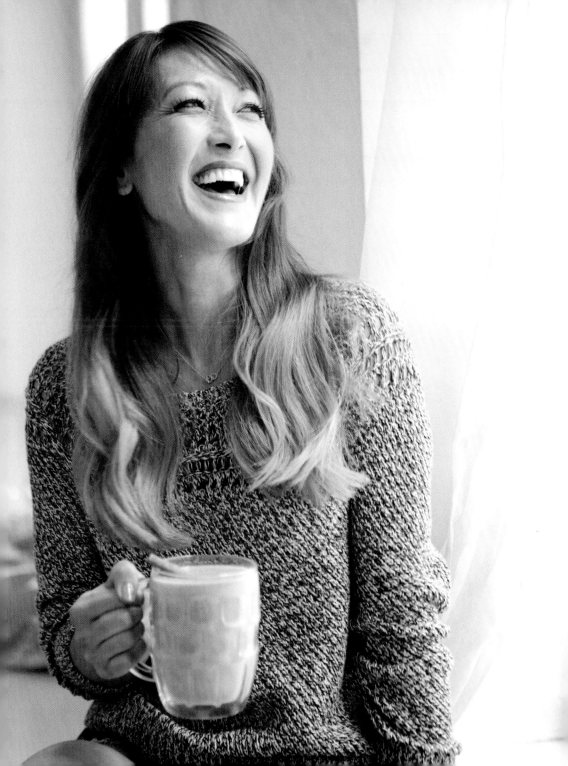

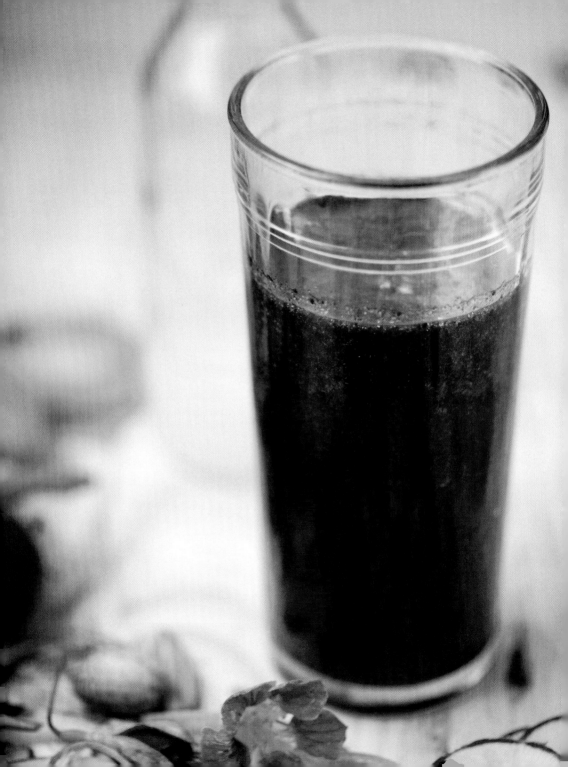

THE CUCUMBER-WATERMELON SKIN CLEANSER

SMOOTHIE › CUCUMBER, WATERMELON

1 cup coconut water

1 cucumber

2 cups watermelon

1 cup ice

Add ingredients into a blender and blend until smooth.

Hydrating your skin from the inside, this cleanser may be your new secret weapon for fighting wrinkles and fine lines. Remember, prevention is key, and going green will keep you glowing strong. #Cleanse

SERVES 2 ▶ **PER SERVING** 60 CALORIES | 0 G FAT | 1 G PROTEIN | 16 G CARBOHYDRATES | 1 G FIBER | 13 G SUGAR | 300 MG POTASSIUM

THE LEMON-BLUEBERRY BLISS

SMOOTHIE › BABY SPINACH, PEAR, BLUEBERRY, LEMON

1 cup coconut water

1 cup organic baby spinach

1 Bartlett pear, halved, cored

2 cups frozen blueberries

2 tablespoons lemon juice

1 teaspoon lemon zest

Add ingredients into a blender and blend until smooth.

Some things just go better together. Like blueberries and lemons. The natural acidity from the lemon will make these beautiful blueberries pop! Not to mention blueberries and all of their healthy glory. See page 30 for more on these beautiful antioxidant-filled bundles!

SERVES 4 ▶ **PER SERVING** 100 CALORIES | 1 G FAT | 1 G PROTEIN | 25 G CARBOHYDRATES | 5 G FIBER | 17 G SUGAR | 280 MG POTASSIUM

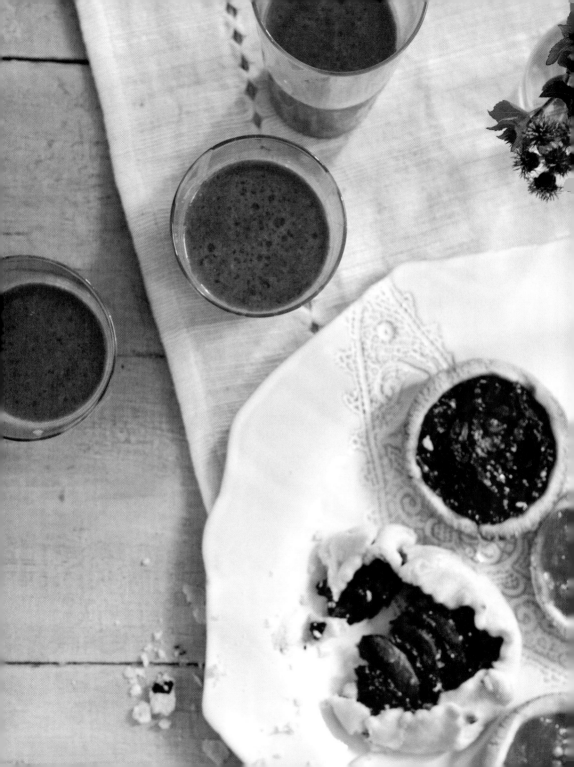

THE COCONUT CUCUMBER PEAR

SMOOTHIE › BABY SPINACH, PEAR, CUCUMBER, COCONUT

1 cup unsweetened
   coconut milk beverage

1 cup baby spinach

1 Bartlett pear, cored

½ large cucumber

1 tablespoon shredded,
   sweetened coconut
   (optional)

1 cup ice

Add ingredients into a blender
and blend until smooth.

Love the skin you have and take good care of it. Skin needs major natural hydration, so drink more water and quench your thirst with this hydrating combination! #CleanGreen.

SERVES 2 ▶ **PER SERVING** 60 CALORIES | 1.5 G FAT | 1 G PROTEIN | 12 G CARBOHYDRATES | 3 G FIBER | 7 G SUGAR | 10% DV VITAMIN D

THE RASPBERRY BEAUTY ELIXIR

SMOOTHIE › BABY SPINACH, RASPBERRY, LAVENDER, RESVERATROL

1½ cups coconut water

2 cups baby spinach

1 cup organic frozen
   raspberries

1 teaspoon fresh lavender
   (or ¼ teaspoon dried)

2 tablespoons resveratrol

1 cup ice

Add ingredients into a blender
and blend until smooth.

Love your beautiful skin, love your girlfriends, and love spa days? Combine all three for a spa-cuisine weekend with the girls. Prepare some delicious treats, decorate with some gorgeous floral arrangements, and blend up some goodness. All the gossip and catch-up will follow naturally. Cheers!

SERVES 2 ▶ **PER SERVING** 70 CALORIES | 0 G FAT | 1 G PROTEIN | 17 G CARBOHYDRATES | 4 G FIBER | 8 G SUGAR | 430 MG POTASSIUM

THE CREAMY CUCUMBER CLEANSER

SMOOTHIE › CUCUMBER, PEAR, MINT

½ cup coconut water

1 cup coconut-almond milk blend

1 medium cucumber, sliced

½ Bartlett pear, cored

3 tablespoons fresh mint

1½ cups ice

Add ingredients into a blender and blend until smooth.

This luscious combination of coconut-almond milk, cucumber, pear, and mint is the kind of "cleansing" you should give your body at least once a week! Cleanse thy life, body, and mind.

SERVES 3 ▶ **PER SERVING** 40 CALORIES | 0.5 G FAT | 1 G PROTEIN | 7 G CARBOHYDRATES | 2 G FIBER | 5 G SUGAR | 15% DV CALCIUM | 15% DV VITAMIN E

THE CREAMY AVOCADO MANGO

SMOOTHIE › ORANGE, BABY SPINACH, AVOCADO, PINEAPPLE, MANGO

1 cup water

1 orange, peeled

2 cups baby spinach

1 ripe avocado, peeled and seeded

½ cup fresh pineapple

1 cup frozen mango

Add ingredients into a blender and blend until smooth.

This delicious, vitamin C-filled, skin-friendly juice is the perfect way to get a rush of nutrients into your body! Cheers to you and that Creamy Avocado glow!

SERVES 4 ▶ **PER SERVING** 140 CALORIES | 7 G FAT | 2 G PROTEIN | 20 G CARBOHYDRATES | 6 G FIBER | 12 G SUGAR | 80% DV VITAMIN C | 15% DV FOLATE

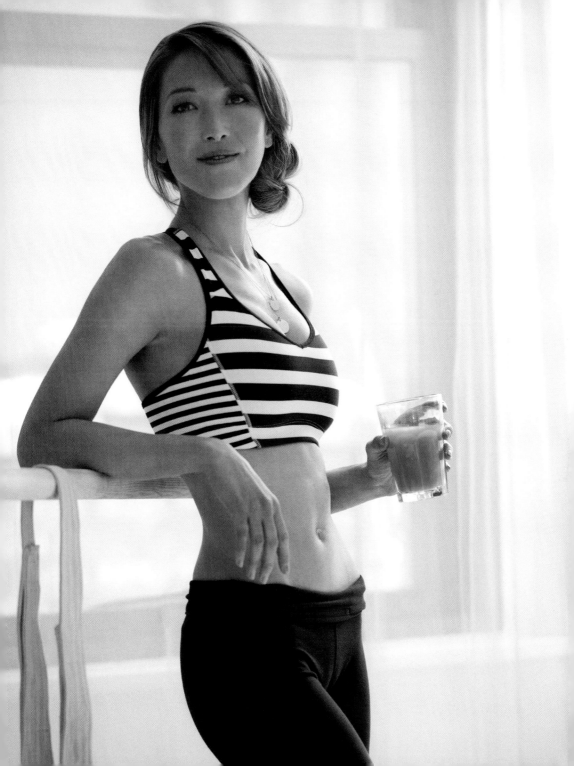

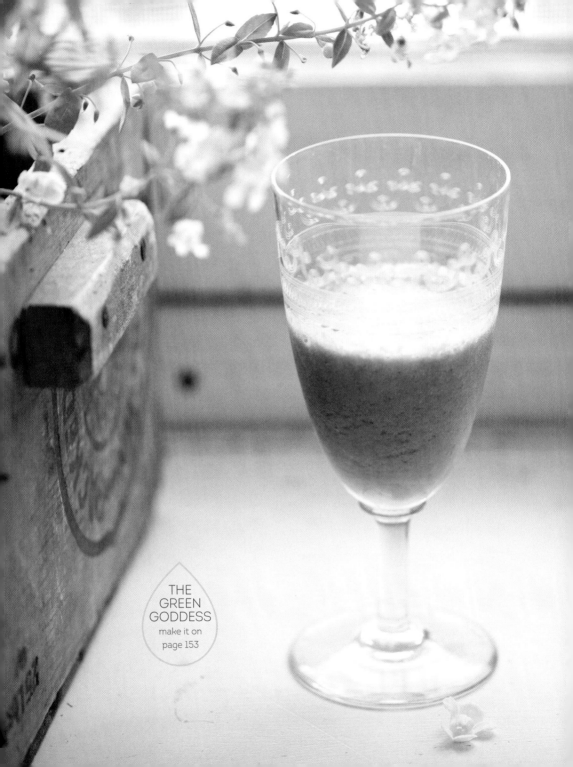

THE
GREEN
GODDESS
make it on
page 153

> "It is not the strongest of the species that survives, nor the most intelligent that survives. It is the one that is the most adaptable to change." *—CHARLES DARWIN*

9

Superfood Brain–Boosting Smoothies

WHO DOESN'T WANT to have optimal brain function going on up there? I am enamored with those who are full of knowledge and who plan to acquire more and more. We must not think that we are above learning once we leave class, for we are creatures of intelligence. Here are some super brain-boosting drinks that certainly can't hurt. Similar to what Charles Darwin found: Create change and you shall survive! Live well.

THE ROMAINE COCONUT

SMOOTHIE › ROMAINE, BANANA, ALMOND BUTTER, COCONUT, FLAXSEED

2 cups unsweetened coconut milk beverage

1 cup romaine lettuce

1 frozen banana

2 tablespoons almond butter

1 tablespoon sweetened coconut shavings

1 tablespoon flaxseed meal

2 teaspoons organic vanilla extract

1 cup ice

Add ingredients into a blender and blend until smooth.

Romaine plus coconut? Yes! This unexpected yet delicious pair blends perfectly, with a touch of flaxseed, for a delightful omega-3 brain boost. Enjoy, smarty.

SERVES 4 ▶ **PER SERVING** 130 CALORIES | 8 G FAT | 3 G PROTEIN | 11 G CARBOHYDRATES | 3 G FIBER | 5 G SUGAR | 15% DV VITAMIN D | 10% DV VITAMIN E | 10% DV FOLATE

"Beauty always starts from the inside. Spread the word." *−CK*

THE GREEN COCONUT ALMOND

SMOOTHIE › BABY SPINACH, GREEN SUPERFOOD, ALMOND BUTTER, HEMP SEED

1 cup unsweetened
coconut milk drink

2 cups baby spinach

2 tablespoons green
superfood

2 tablespoons almond
butter

¼ teaspoon cinnamon

1 tablespoon hemp seed

1 cup ice

Add ingredients into a blender
and blend until smooth.

Almond butter is one of my absolute favorite treats.
With two delightful scoops of it, a bunch of spinach,
hemp seed, and cinnamon, this Green Coconut
Almond smoothie is a perfect blend for a brain boost
that can also make you sound really, really cool.

SERVES 2 ▶ **PER SERVING** 240 CALORIES | 15 G FAT | 10 G PROTEIN |
16 G CARBOHYDRATES | 8 G FIBER | 3 G SUGAR | 35% DV CALCIUM |
80% DV IRON | 20% DV VITAMIN E

THE GREEN GODDESS

SMOOTHIE › BABY SPINACH, PINEAPPLE, CUCUMBER, FLAXSEED, PROTEIN POWDER

1½ cups unsweetened
almond milk

2 cups baby spinach

2 cups kale

1½ cups pineapple

1 large cucumber

1 tablespoon ground
flaxseed

4 tablespoons (1 scoop)
protein powder

2 cups ice

Add ingredients into a blender
and blend until smooth.

With fresh pineapple and brain-boosting flaxseed,
this delicious-detoxing beverage will have you
looking like a goddess and feeling like a beauty
queen (or king)!

SERVES 4 ▶ **PER SERVING** 130 CALORIES | 3 G FAT | 9 G PROTEIN |
17 G CARBOHYDRATES | 4 G FIBER | 7 G SUGAR | 420 MG POTASSIUM |
80% DV VITAMIN A | 120% DV VITAMIN C

THE CH-CH-CH CHIA!

SMOOTHIE › BABY SPINACH, BANANA, ALMOND BUTTER, CHIA SEED

1½ cups unsweetened
   coconut milk beverage

3 cups baby spinach

1 frozen banana

2 tablespoons almond
   butter

3 tablespoons chia seeds

2 teaspoons organic
   vanilla extract

½ cup ice

Add ingredients into a blender
and blend until smooth.

To keep your brain sharp and your mind calm, chia seeds are a great Clean Green ingredient, with omega-3 fatty acids, antioxidants, fiber, protein, and phosphorus—all natural nutrients to keep your body happy!

SERVES 2 ▶ **PER SERVING** 190 CALORIES | 11 G FAT | 5 G PROTEIN | 19 G CARBOHYDRATES | 7 G FIBER | 6 G SUGAR | 1,880 MG OMEGA-3 | 15% DV VITAMIN D | 8% DV FOLATE

THE DARK CHOCOLATE CHIA

SMOOTHIE › KALE, BANANA, DATES, CHIA SEED, CHOCOLATE

1¼ cups unsweetened
   almond milk

2 cups kale

1 frozen banana

2 dried dates, pitted

2 tablespoons chia seeds

2 tablespoons unpro-
   cessed, unsweetened
   cocoa powder

1 cup ice

Add ingredients into a blender
and blend until smooth.

With feel-good chemicals and anti-aging benefits, you bet your ass that dark chocolate/cocoa powder plays a part in this book. Add in some more spirulina or green superfood to this one for an extra boost of goodness.

SERVES 2 ▶ **PER SERVING** 130 CALORIES | 4.5 G FAT | 5 G PROTEIN | 22 G CARBOHYDRATES | 6 G FIBER | 8 G SUGAR | 1,340 MG OMEGA-3 | 100% DV VITAMIN C | 20% DV CALCIUM

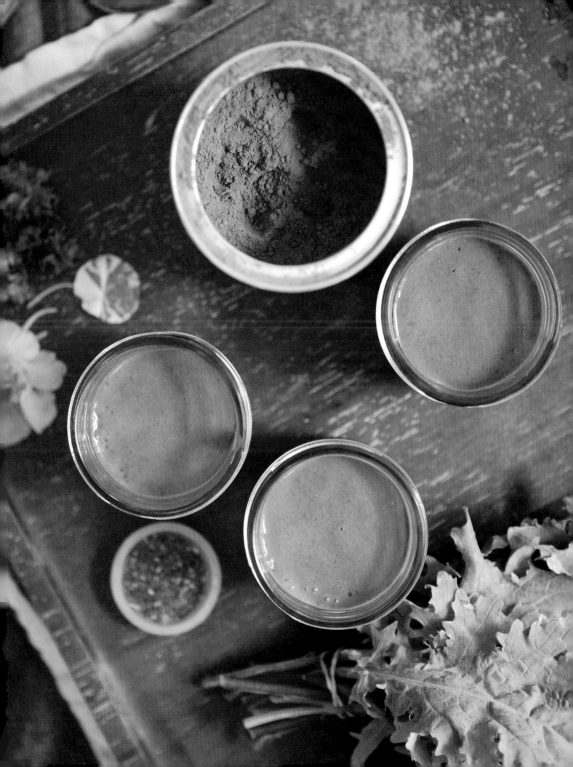

THE CREAMY GREEN AVOCADO-PEACH

SMOOTHIE ❯ BABY SPINACH, PEACH, FLAXSEED, AVOCADO

- 1 **cup unsweetened almond milk**
- 2 **cups baby spinach**
- 2 **cups frozen organic peaches**
- 1 **teaspoon flaxseed oil**
- 1 **ripe avocado, pitted**

Add ingredients into a blender and blend until smooth.

With its creamy texture and healthy monounsaturated fat content, avocado also gives your blood a healthy rush. Get glowin'!

SERVES 4 ▶ **PER SERVING** 190 CALORIES : 14 G FAT : 3 G PROTEIN : 17 G CARBOHYDRATES : 7 G FIBER : 8 G SUGAR : 1,700 MG OMEGA-3 : 150% DV VITAMIN C : 15% DV FOLATE

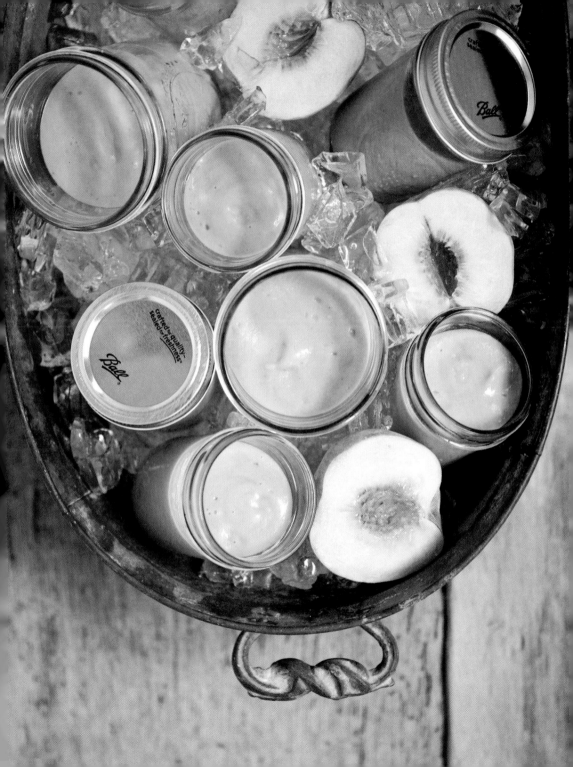

THE GREEN ALMOND PUMPKIN

SMOOTHIE ❯ BABY SPINACH, PUMPKIN PUREE, FLAXSEED, ALMOND BUTTER

1 **cup unsweetened almond milk**

2 **cups baby spinach**

¾ **cup organic pumpkin puree**

2 **tablespoons flaxseed meal**

2 **tablespoons almond butter**

½ **teaspoon pumpkin spice**

1 **cup ice (optional)**

Add ingredients into a blender and blend until smooth.

Almond butter (full of healthy fats), pumpkin puree, flaxseed meal, and a dash of pumpkin spice come together here for a pleasantly surprising brain boost in a glass. For an even bigger brain bonus, add in a touch of flax or hempseed oil.

SERVES 2 ▶ **PER SERVING** 190 CALORIES | 13 G FAT
7 G PROTEIN | 16 G CARBOHYDRATES | 9 G FIBER | 4 G SUGAR
1,200 MG OMEGA-3 | 250% DV VITAMIN A | 45% DV VITAMIN E

THE GREEN DATE "SHAKE"

SMOOTHIE ❯ BABY SPINACH, KALE, BANANA, DATES, CHIA SEED, FLAXSEED

1 **cup unsweetened almond milk**

2 **cups baby spinach**

1 **cup kale**

1 **frozen banana**

3 **dried dates, pitted**

1 **tablespoon chia seeds**

1 **teaspoon flaxseed oil**

1 **tablespoon organic vanilla extract**

Add ingredients into a blender and blend until smooth.

This delicious "shake" contains chia seeds and flaxseed oil, which both lead to better brain power.

SERVES 2 ▶ **PER SERVING** 190 CALORIES | 6 G FAT
4 G PROTEIN | 31 G CARBOHYDRATES | 7 G FIBER | 15 G SUGAR
2,200 MG OMEGA-3 | 90% DV VITAMIN A | 80% DV VITAMIN C

THE CLEAN GREEN TEA

SMOOTHIE › BABY SPINACH, KALE, BANANA, MATCHA

1¼ cups unsweetened
almond milk

1 cup baby spinach

1 cup kale

1 frozen banana

2 teaspoons matcha green
tea powder

1 tablespoon chia seeds

1 teaspoon flaxseed oil

1 teaspoon maple syrup
(optional)

½ cup ice (optional)

Add ingredients into a
blender and blend until
smooth.

This Japanese green tea–inspired smoothie not only tastes like green tea ice cream, it plays an important role in enhancing your brain's function. Drink to optimum health and wellness the Clean Green way.

SERVES 2 ▶ **PER SERVING** 150 CALORIES | 6 G FAT | 4 G PROTEIN | 22 G CARBOHYDRATES | 5 G FIBER | 8 G SUGAR | 2,200 MG OMEGA-3 | 80% DV VITAMIN A | 80% DV VITAMIN C | 35% DV VITAMIN E

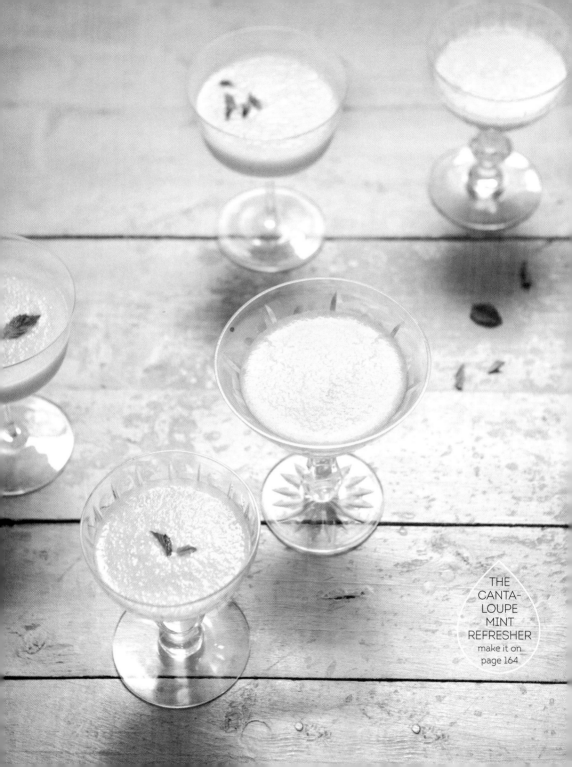

THE
CANTA-
LOUPE
MINT
REFRESHER
make it on
page 164

10

"Peace, love, and green juice." —CK

Happy, Flat Tummy Juices & Smoothies

WE ALL WANT one, and we can absolutely have one—a flat belly! To soothe and aid in digestion, these drinks were created to help calm your tummy. Test a few out with extra ginger, fresh mint, and/or parsley—all ingredients that help comfort (and even flatten) your tummy, the organic way.

THE GREEN CUCUMBER CLEANSER

1 large cucumber

¼ Fuji or Granny Smith apple

¼ cup fresh parsley

1 tablespoon lemon juice (optional)

Juice all ingredients into a glass; whisk in lemon juice.

This happy-tummy juice helps to soothe naturally with cucumber, apple, fresh parsley, and lemon. Watch out: Green juice is the new de-bloat on the block.

SERVES 1 ▶ **PER SERVING** 45 CALORIES 0.5 G FAT 2 G PROTEIN 9 G CARBOHYDRATES 0 G FIBER 8 G SUGAR 490 MG POTASSIUM 25% DV VITAMIN A 50% DV VITAMIN C

THE GREEN PINEAPPLE

SMOOTHIE › BABY SPINACH, PINEAPPLE

1 cup unsweetened almond milk

3 cups baby spinach

1 cup fresh pineapple (or frozen pineapple)

1 cup ice

Add ingredients into a blender and blend until smooth.

Pineapple can help prevent tummy bloat with its natural digestive enzymes. It also boasts bromelain, which contains anti-inflammatory properties and may also help increase blood circulation. Hell, yeah! Let's hear it for pineapple!

SERVES 2-4 ▶ **PER SERVING** 80 CALORIES 1.5 G FAT 2 G PROTEIN 16 G CARBOHYDRATES 3 G FIBER 8 G SUGAR 70% DV VITAMIN C 10% DV VITAMIN D 25% DV VITAMIN E

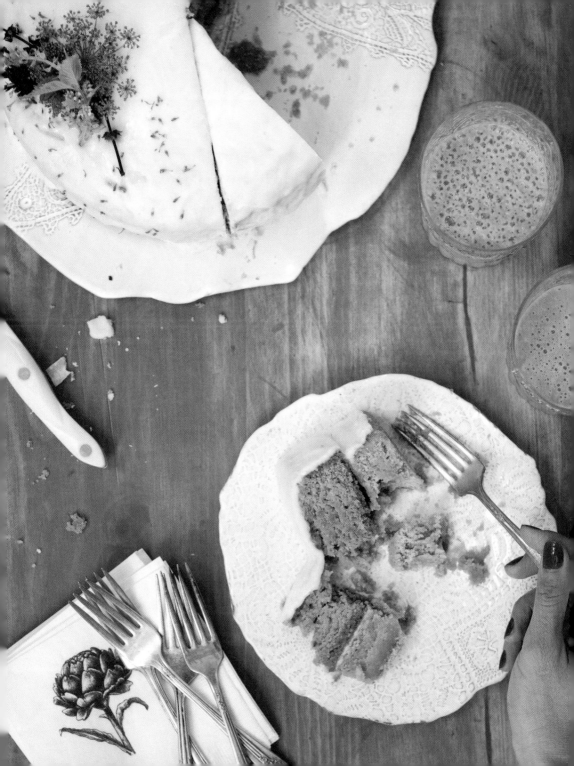

THE CANTALOUPE MINT REFRESHER

SMOOTHIE > CANTALOUPE, MINT

1 cup unsweetened almond milk

2 cups cantaloupe melon

3 tablespoons fresh mint

1 cup ice

Add ingredients into a blender and blend until smooth.

This delicious blend of cantaloupe, soothing fresh mint, and a hint of almond milk will sing to your happy, flat tummy.

SERVES 3 ▶ **PER SERVING** 45 CALORIES | 1 G FAT | 1 G PROTEIN | 8 G CARBOHYDRATES | 0 G FIBER | 8 G SUGAR | 80% DV VITAMIN A | 8% DV VITAMIN D | 15% DV VITAMIN E

THE GINGER-VANILLA DETOX

SMOOTHIE > BANANA, PEAR, GINGER, YOGURT

1 cup unsweetened almond milk

1 frozen banana

½ pear

1 tablespoon fresh ginger, grated

1 teaspoon organic vanilla extract

½ cup Greek or coconut yogurt

1½ cups ice

Add ingredients into a blender and blend until smooth.

I developed this juice with all of my spa days in mind. With notes of pear, fresh ginger for the tummy, and yummy Greek yogurt to soothe, this detoxifying blend can keep you Zen, calm, and feeling good about what you're consuming.

SERVES 3 ▶ **PER SERVING** 90 CALORIES | 1 G FAT | 4 G PROTEIN | 16 G CARBOHYDRATES | 2 G FIBER | 9 G SUGAR | 10% DV CALCIUM | 8% DV VITAMIN D | 15% DV VITAMIN E

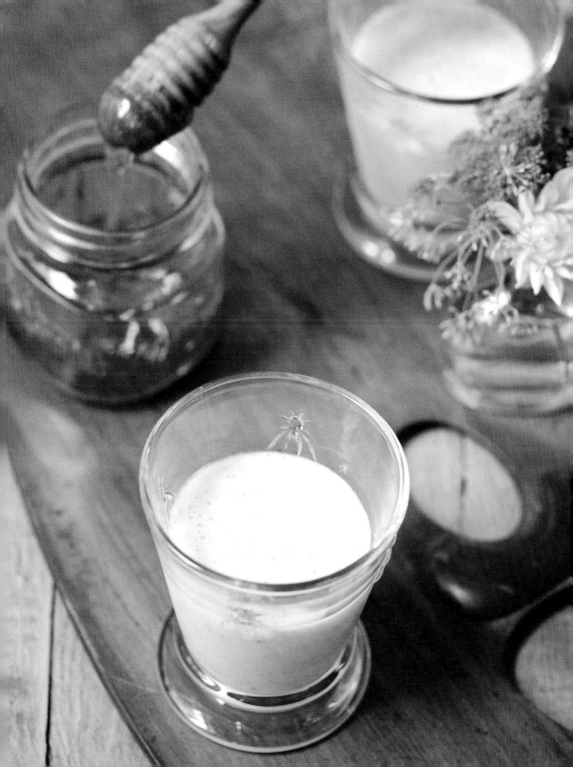

THE GREEN PEACH
SMOOTHIE › BABY SPINACH, PEACH, PEAR, GREEN SUPERFOOD

1½ cups unsweetened
   almond milk

2 cups baby spinach

2 cups frozen, organic
   peaches

½ Bartlett pear, cored

1 teaspoon bee pollen
   (optional)

1 tablespoon green
   superfood

Add ingredients into a blender
and blend until smooth.

Creamy organic peaches blended with spinach and green superfood make for a delicious and supremely satisfying way to relax, recharge, and flatten that belly on the weekends! Reboot your battery on Saturday and Sunday! Debauchery is so 10 years ago.

SERVES 4 ▶ **PER SERVING** 100 CALORIES | 1.5 G FAT |
3 G PROTEIN | 19 G CARBOHYDRATES | 5 G FIBER | 11 G SUGAR |
150% DV VITAMIN C | 25% DV IRON | 25% DV VITAMIN E

THE SWEET GREEN APPLE
JUICE › BABY SPINACH, KALE, CUCUMBER, PINEAPPLE, APPLE

3 cups baby spinach

2 cups kale

2 medium cucumbers

½ cup fresh pineapple

1 Fuji apple

Add all ingredients into a
juicer and juice.

With crisp Fuji apples, deliciously fresh cucumbers, and of course, our green friends kale and spinach, this juice will have you feeling cleansed and calm with a content tummy in mind.

SERVES 2 ▶ **PER SERVING** 100 CALORIES | 1 G FAT | 5 G PROTEIN |
22 G CARBOHYDRATES | 0 G FIBER | 15 G SUGAR | 730 MG POTASSIUM |
160% DV VITAMIN A | 190% DV VITAMIN C | 15% DV CALCIUM

166

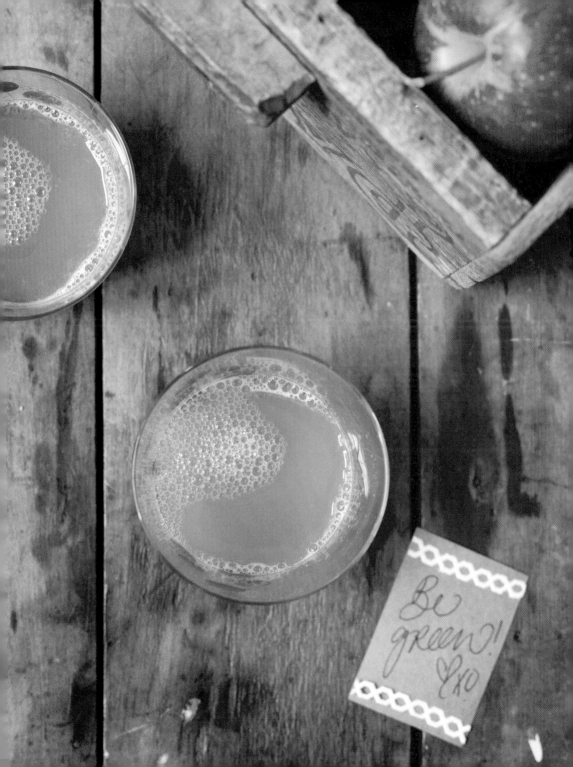

THE PUMPKIN PEAR

SMOOTHIE > BABY SPINACH, PEAR, PINEAPPLE, PUMPKIN PUREE

1½ cups unsweetened coconut almond milk

2 cups baby spinach

1 Bartlett pear, cored

¾ cup fresh pineapple

¾ cup organic pumpkin puree

¼ teaspoon pumpkin spice

1 cup ice

Add ingredients into a blender and blend until smooth.

This duo of pumpkin and pear is a perfect match of feel-good foods. Pumpkin spice is full of benefits, such as improving colon health and digestion, and even has anti-inflammatory benefits.

SERVES 4 ▶ **PER SERVING** 80 CALORIES | 1.5 G FAT | 2 G PROTEIN | 16 G CARBOHYDRATES | 5 G FIBER | 9 G SUGAR | 130% DV VITAMIN A | 10% DV CALCIUM | 20% DV VITAMIN E

THE GRAPEFRUIT SOOTHER

JUICE > CARROT, CUCUMBER, GRAPEFRUIT, GINGER

4 organic carrots, scrubbed

½ large cucumber

1 pink grapefruit, peeled

1 teaspoon ginger

Add all ingredients into a juicer and juice.

While having a "moment" on set (you know, PMS, bloating, unhappy tummy), I had to come up with something to calm my tummy quickly. I combined grapefruit and ginger to save the day; 20 minutes and two glasses later, I was back to a good ol' happy disposition. Enjoy, my lovely. Soothe that belly!

SERVES 1 ▶ **PER SERVING** 160 CALORIES | 1 G FAT | 4 G PROTEIN | 37 G CARBOHYDRATES | 0 G FIBER | 13 G SUGAR | 1,290 MG POTASSIUM | 830% DV VITAMIN A | 160% DV VITAMIN C | 15% DV FOLATE

THE GREEN CARROT GINGER

JUICE › BABY SPINACH, CARROT, PEAR, GINGER

5 cups baby spinach

3 organic carrots, scrubbed

½ Bartlett pear, cored

1 tablespoon ginger

Add all ingredients into a juicer and juice.

This delicious trifecta of spinach, carrots, and ginger will have your tummy soothed and your cells feeling revitalized. No need for that chemical-laden energy drink. Spinach has always had all the answers.

SERVES 1 ▶ **PER SERVING** | 120 CALORIES | 0.5 G FAT | 5 G PROTEIN | 25 G CARBOHYDRATES | 0 G FIBER | 17 G SUGAR | 700% DV VITAMIN A | 25% DV IRON | 10% DV FOLATE

LE PEACH KALE

JUICE › KALE, BABY SPINACH, PEACH, CUCUMBER

1 cup kale

4 cups baby spinach

¾ fresh peach, pitted

½ medium cucumber

Add all ingredients into a juicer and juice.

Juicy, fresh peach, spinach, and cucumber all lead to one gorgeous, green, lean, and clean juice. Just do it. Le Peach Kale.

SERVES 1 ▶ **PER SERVING** | 90 CALORIES | 1 G FAT | 6 G PROTEIN | 16 G CARBOHYDRATES | 0 G FIBER | 10 G SUGAR | 210% DV VITAMIN A | 180% DV VITAMIN C | 25% DV CALCIUM

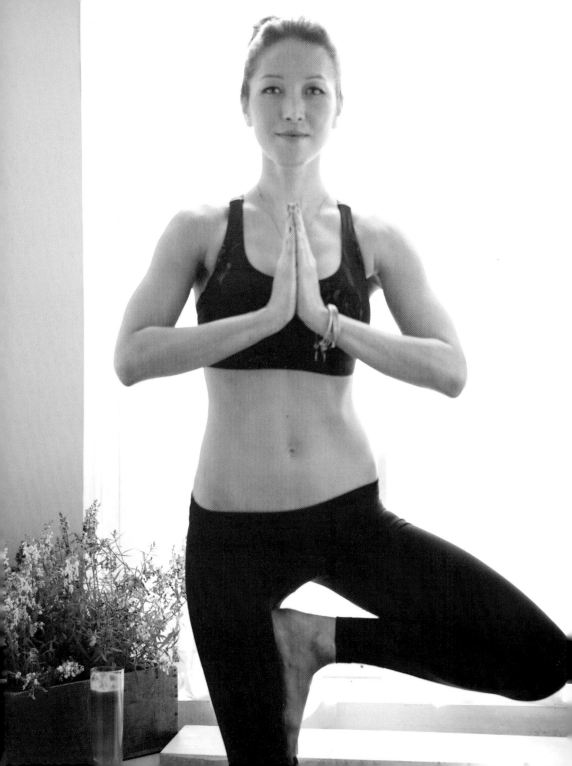

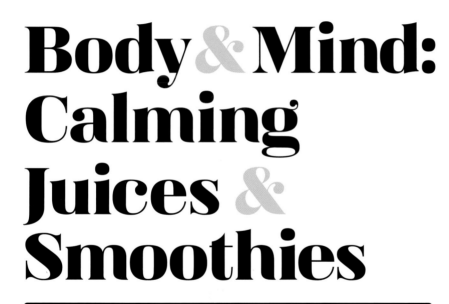

"What we are today comes from our thoughts of yesterday, and our present thoughts build our life of tomorrow: Our life is the creation of our mind."

–*BUDDHA (SIDDHARTHA GAUTAMA)*

11

Body & Mind: Calming Juices & Smoothies

EVER GET INTO one of those moods that you can't kick? I've found a simple solution for you: good music, meditation, and a green juice in your hand. Here are 12 delicious Clean Green ways to relax and enjoy a calming beverage during a moment of stress. Because we ALL have those moments. Deep breaths. #CleanGreenExhale

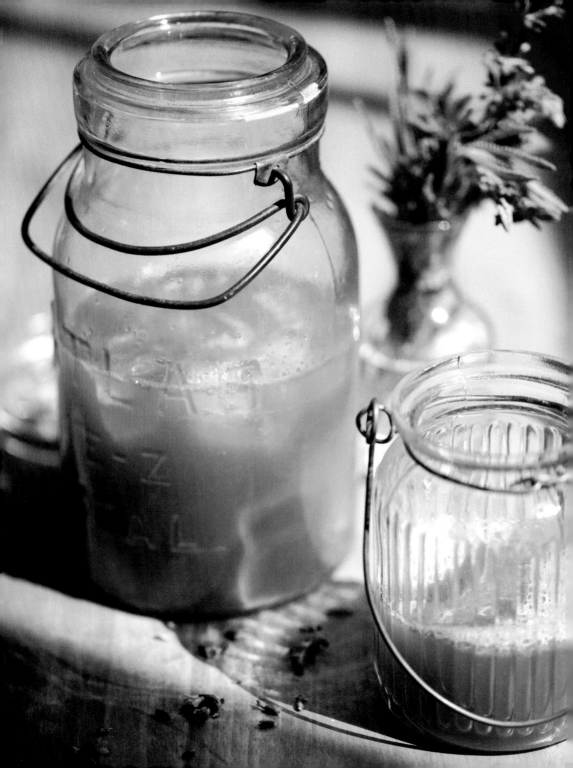

THE LAVENDER-MELON REFRESHER

JUICE > BABY SPINACH, MELON, LAVENDER

3 cups baby spinach

1 cup honeydew melon

2 tablespoons fresh lavender

1 cup coconut water

½ cup water

Juice spinach, melon, and lavender into a glass. Add the coconut water and whisk well to combine.

I absolutely love juicing with lavender. I find its soothing aromatic properties really help me relax and stay calm through the storm of working in New York City. Keep a lavender plant at your desk or by your window for those moments of need or for emergency juicing!

SERVES 2 ▶ **PER SERVING** 60 CALORIES | 0 G FAT | 2 G PROTEIN | 13 G CARBOHYDRATES | 0 G FIBER | 11 G SUGAR | 500 MG POTASSIUM | 30% DV VITAMIN A | 35% DV VITAMIN C | 20% DV IRON

THE LAVENDER CUCUMBER BLEND

SMOOTHIE › CUCUMBER, LAVENDER, YOGURT, MINT

1 cup unsweetened almond milk

1 cucumber

1 tablespoon fresh lavender (or 1 teaspoon dried)

1 cup Greek or coconut yogurt

1 tablespoon mint

1 cup ice

Add ingredients into a blender and blend until smooth.

For a relaxed and calm mind, try the Clean Green Lavender Cucumber Blend. A delicious, sweet, and fab treat, try out this smoothie with a face mask, a nail polish change, and a best friend.

SERVES 2 ▶ **PER SERVING** 70 CALORIES | 1 G FAT | 8 G PROTEIN | 7 G CARBOHYDRATES | 1 G FIBER | 5 G SUGAR | 15% DV CALCIUM | 8% DV VITAMIN D | 15% DV VITAMIN E

THE BASIL MELON DETOX

JUICE › HONEYDEW MELON, BABY SPINACH, BASIL, MINT, CUCUMBER

1 cup honeydew melon

3 cups baby spinach

¼ cup fresh basil

¼ cup fresh mint

1 large cucumber

Add all ingredients into a juicer and juice.

Refreshing basil, honeydew melon, and fresh mint will have you juicing this trifecta of freshness at your next Sunday brunch. Impressive party favor? You bet! And your guests are totally worth it!

SERVES 2 ▶ **PER SERVING** 45 CALORIES | 0 G FAT | 2 G PROTEIN | 10 G CARBOHYDRATES | 0 G FIBER | 9 G SUGAR | 35% DV VITAMIN A | 45% DV VITAMIN C | 10% DV IRON

THE CALM MELON

½ cup coconut water

1 cup honeydew melon

2 cups baby spinach

2 tablespoons fresh mint

1 teaspoon fresh lavender

1 cup ice

Add ingredients into a blender and blend until smooth.

Sometimes we all just need a moment of Zen. This is my calming melon-and-mint way to chill out over a long weekend. Be calm and green. Just be.

SERVES 3 ▶ **PER SERVING** 50 CALORIES | 0 G FAT | 1 G PROTEIN | 13 G CARBOHYDRATES | 2 G FIBER | 9 G SUGAR | 20% DV VITAMIN A | 30% DV VITAMIN C | 6% DV IRON

THE M4: MINT-MELON-MANGO MOOD BOOSTER

1 cup coconut water

1 cup frozen mango

2 cups baby spinach

1 cup honeydew melon

¼ cup fresh mint

1½ cups ice

Add ingredients into a blender and blend until smooth.

The M4: Not just a hot car. This Mint, Melon, Mango Mood Booster is a refreshing summer-like treat. With calming notes from the melon and mint, you'll be feeling like sunshine in no time!

SERVES 3 ▶ **PER SERVING** 80 CALORIES | 0 G FAT | 1 G PROTEIN | 21 G CARBOHYDRATES | 3 G FIBER | 17 G SUGAR | 25% DV VITAMIN A | 50% DV VITAMIN C | 4% DV FOLATE

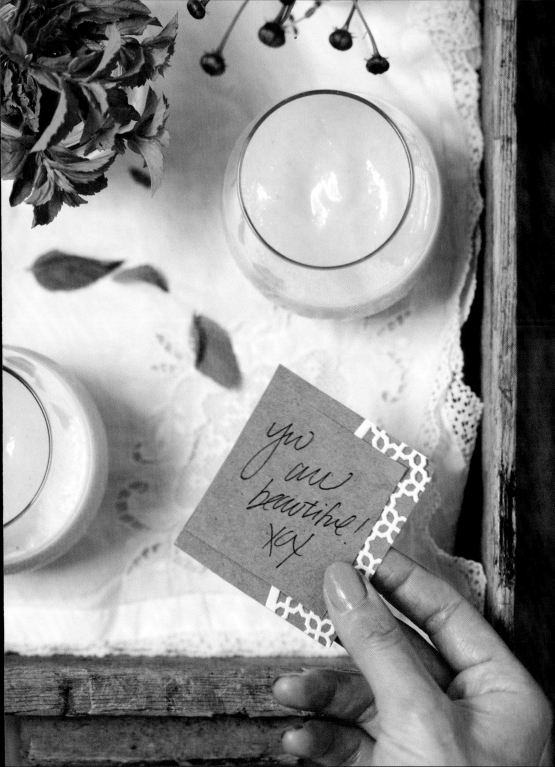

THE CHOCOLATE
AVOCADO GODDESS

SMOOTHIE ⟩ AVOCADO, BANANA, CHOCOLATE

1¼ cups unsweetened almond milk

1 ripe avocado, pitted

1 frozen banana

2 tablespoons dark unsweetened cocoa powder

2 teaspoons agave nectar (if you must)

1 cup ice

Add ingredients into a blender and blend until smooth.

With creamy and luscious avocado and dark cocoa powder, this Chocolate Avocado Goddess is the favorite of many of my powerhouse publicist and news anchor girlfriends on the go in NYC. They're proof the recipe works! #Chocolatefix

SERVES 2 ▶ **PER SERVING** 180 CALORIES | 12 G FAT | 3 G PROTEIN | 21 G CARBOHYDRATES | 7 G FIBER | 9 G SUGAR | 600 MG POTASSIUM | 10% DV CALCIUM | 10% DV VITAMIN D | 30% DV VITAMIN E | 15% DV FOLATE

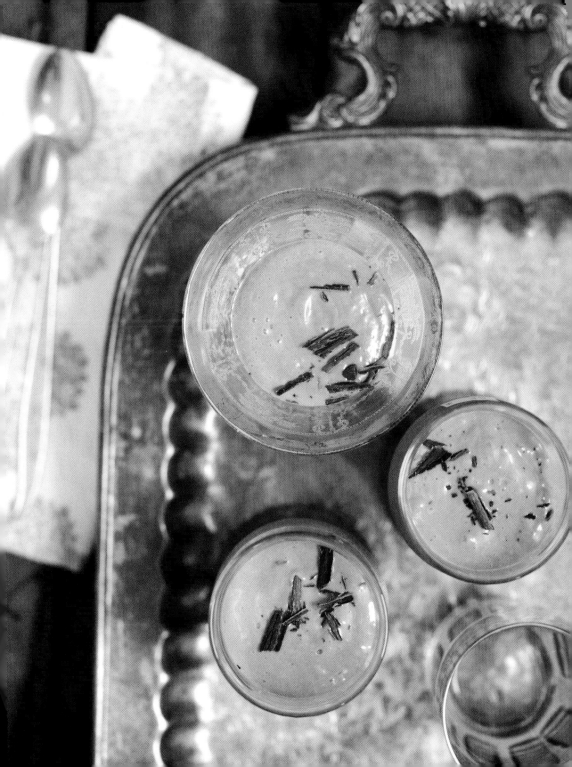

THE VANILLA-PEAR "SHAKE"

SMOOTHIE > BANANA, PEAR, VANILLA

1 **cup unsweetened almond milk**

1 **frozen banana**

1 **Bartlett pear, cored**

1 **tablespoon organic vanilla extract**

1 **cup ice**

Add ingredients into a blender and blend until smooth.

With organic vanilla and sweet pears, this delicious beverage is perfect for a calming dessert at the end of the day. Sure, you can green-drink for dessert! You look gorgeous when you relax.

SERVES 2 ▶ **PER SERVING** 150 CALORIES : 2 G FAT : 1 G PROTEIN : 29 G CARBOHYDRATES : 5 G FIBER : 17 G SUGAR : 410 MG POTASSIUM : 10% DV CALCIUM : 10% DV VITAMIN D : 25% DV VITAMIN E

THE LAVENDER BLUEBERRY

SMOOTHIE > KALE, BANANA, BLUEBERRY, LAVENDER

2 **cups unsweetened almond milk**

2 **cups kale**

1 **frozen banana**

1 **cup frozen blueberries**

1 **tablespoon fresh lavender (or 1 teaspoon dried lavender)**

1 **teaspoon bee pollen**

1 **tablespoon green superfood**

Add ingredients into a blender and blend until smooth.

One of my favorite combinations, this lavender and blueberry treat brings bliss to the table. Serve it up for a Clean Green dinner or share it for a Zen-like dessert.

SERVES 4 ▶ **PER SERVING** 100 CALORIES : 2.5 G FAT : 4 G PROTEIN : 18 G CARBOHYDRATES : 4 G FIBER : 7 G SUGAR : 450 MG POTASSIUM : 80% DV VITAMIN A : 80% DV VITAMIN C : 20% DV IRON : 25% DV VITAMIN E

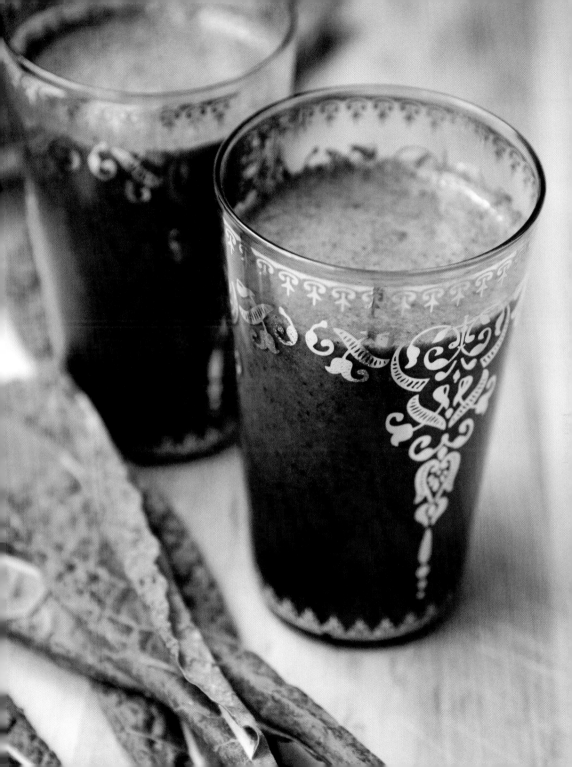

THE HONEYDEW MINT REFRESHER

SMOOTHIE › HONEYDEW MELON, MINT

1 **cup unsweetened coconut-almond milk**

1 **cup honeydew melon**

3 **tablespoons fresh mint leaves**

1 **tablespoon bee pollen**

1 **teaspoon probiotics/ acidophilus**

1½ **cups ice**

Add ingredients into a blender and blend until smooth.

Sweet, refreshing, and delightful, this combination (with a touch of bee pollen) is a perfect refresher and a sweet, minty treat to end your day. Enjoy with a relaxing bath or for a spa weekend with the girls.

SERVES 2 ▶ **PER SERVING** 70 CALORIES ¦ 2 G FAT ¦ 3 G PROTEIN ¦ 12 G CARBOHYDRATES ¦ 2 G FIBER ¦ 7 G SUGAR ¦ 35% DV VITAMIN C ¦ 25% DV CALCIUM ¦ 30% DV VITAMIN E

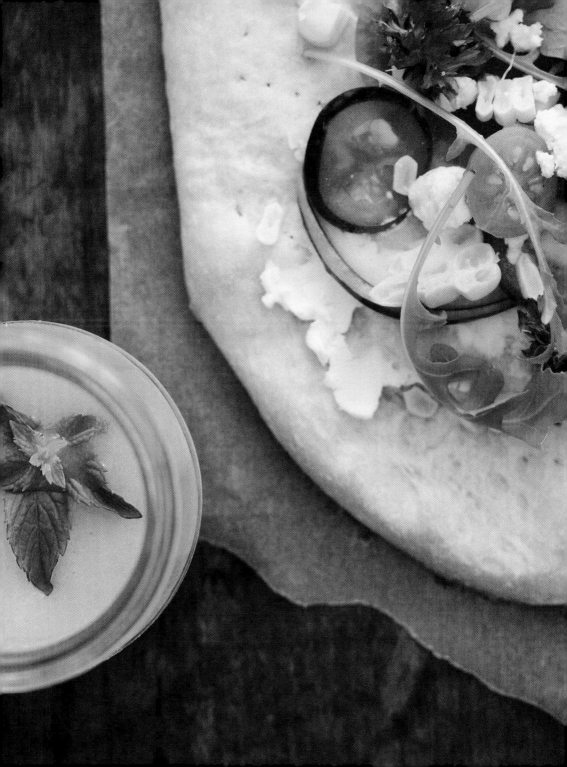

Mood-Boosting Manganese

BLOOD LEVELS OF MANGANESE vary throughout that time of month, so it's not surprising that this mineral might be involved in PMS. Studies suggest that eating manganese-rich foods may reduce the moodiness and irritability associated with "that time of the month." Some Clean Green sources of manganese include: pineapple, spinach, pumpkin seeds, walnuts, oats, quinoa, flax-seed, and raspberries.

THE CALMING GREEN PINEAPPLE

JUICE ▷ BABY SPINACH, CUCUMBER, PINEAPPLE, GINGER

2 cups baby spinach

1 large cucumber

¼ cup fresh pineapple

1 tablespoon fresh ginger

Add all ingredients into a juicer and juice.

For a day of destressing and relaxing by the pool. Try out the Calming Green Pineapple; sip it beach-side or after a yoga session!

SERVES 2 (SMALL GLASSES) ▶ **PER SERVING** 50 CALORIES | 0.5 G FAT | 3 G PROTEIN | 10 G CARBOHYDRATES | 0 G FIBER | 9 G SUGAR | 35% DV VITAMIN A | 60% DV VITAMIN C | 10% DV IRON

THE CHOCOLATE PEANUT BUTTER CUP (TASTES LIKE A MILKSHAKE!)

SMOOTHIE ▶ BABY SPINACH, BANANA, PEANUT BUTTER, CHOCOLATE, PROTEIN POWDER

- 1 cup unsweetened almond milk
- 2 cups baby spinach
- 1 frozen banana
- 2 tablespoons natural peanut butter
- 2 tablespoons unsweetened cocoa powder
- 4 tablespoons (1 scoop) protein powder
- 1 cup ice

Add ingredients into a blender and blend until smooth.

So the drink apparently matches the name. Surprised? I tested this milkshake-like treat for all of you. Enjoy those greens in a whole new way!

SERVES 2 ▶ **PER SERVING** 180 CALORIES | 7 G FAT | 12 G PROTEIN | 17 G CARBOHYDRATES | 4 G FIBER | 6 G SUGAR | 10% DV CALCIUM | 20% DV IRON | 15% DV VITAMIN E

THE CINNAMON PINEAPPLE GREEN

SMOOTHIE ▶ BABY SPINACH, BANANA, PINEAPPLE

- 1½ cups unsweetened coconut-almond milk
- 2 cups baby spinach
- 1 frozen banana
- 1 cup fresh pineapple
- ½ teaspoon cinnamon

Add ingredients into a blender and blend until smooth.

The combination of sweet pineapple and a touch of cinnamon sounds like a fragrant, tropical dream, right? Cinnamon can help ease the mind while pineapple can aid digestion.

SERVES 4 ▶ **PER SERVING** 90 CALORIES | 1.5 G FAT | 2 G PROTEIN | 19 G CARBOHYDRATES | 3 G FIBER | 10 G SUGAR | 50% DV VITAMIN C | 25% DV CALCIUM | 10% DV VITAMIN D | 25% DV VITAMIN E

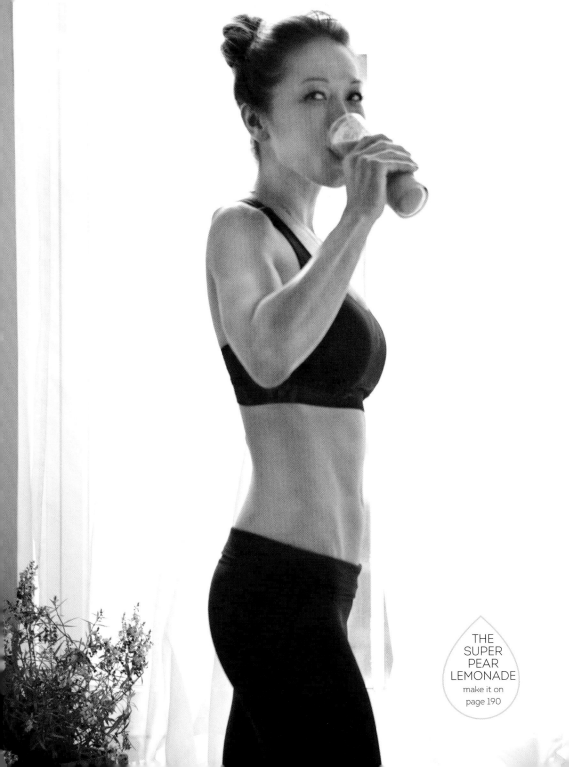

THE
SUPER
PEAR
LEMONADE
make it on
page 190

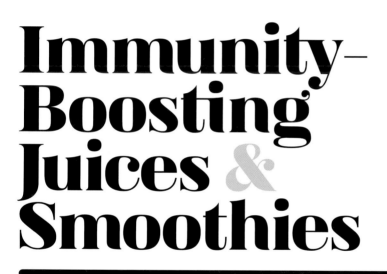

"To ensure good health: Eat lightly, breathe deeply, live moderately, cultivate cheerfulness, and maintain an interest in life."

—WILLIAM LONDEN

12

Immunity–Boosting Juices & Smoothies

WHEN YOU FEEL a cold coming on, I urge you to head to your local market rather than the drugstore. In Western medicine we are so accustomed to "masking," "treating," and "getting better." However, with Japanese medicine, I have learned to focus on prevention. These 11 recipes will do just that.

THE CARROT GINGER

JUICE › CARROT, GINGER, CUCUMBER

1 **pound organic carrots, scrubbed**

1 **tablespoon fresh ginger**

1 **large cucumber**

Add all ingredients into a juicer and juice.

If you love carrot-ginger soup, you will love this delicious combination of sweet and hot! Enjoy this juice alongside a healthy breakfast or with a satisfying Clean Green dinner. You're gorgeous, you carrot-ginge-lover, you.

SERVES 2 ▶ **PER SERVING** 80 CALORIES | 1 G FAT | 3 G PROTEIN | 18 G CARBOHYDRATES | 0 G FIBER | 13 G SUGAR | 930 MG POTASSIUM | 760% DV VITAMIN A | 10% DV CALCIUM | 10% DV FOLATE

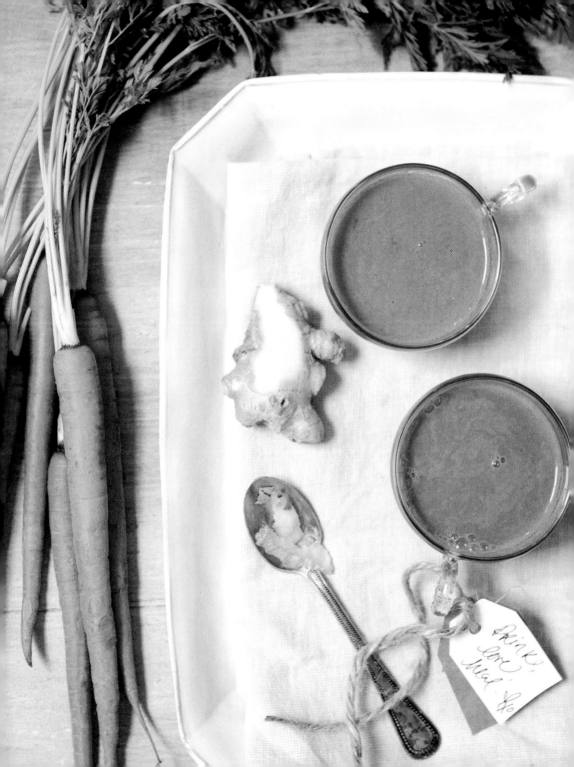

THE SUPER PEAR LEMONADE

JUICE › BABY SPINACH, LEMON, PEAR

3 cups baby spinach

½ lemon

1 Bartlett pear, cored

½ cup coconut water

½ cup water

Juice spinach, lemon, and pear into a glass. Add the coconut water and water, then whisk well to combine.

If you love your lemonade, you're gonna love the kick in this super-tart immunity-boosting pear lemonade. With crisp, fresh baby spinach, sweetness from the pear, and tartness from the lemon, you've got serious "aid" to your health. Cheers.

SERVES 2 ▶ **PER SERVING** 60 CALORIES | 0 G FAT | 1 G PROTEIN | 14 G CARBOHYDRATES | 0 G FIBER | 11 G SUGAR | 220 MG POTASSIUM | 25% DV VITAMIN A | 25% DV VITAMIN C

THE GREEN SUPER-IMMUNITY LEMONADE

JUICE › BABY SPINACH, HONEYDEW MELON, LEMON, CUCUMBER

5 cups baby spinach

1 cup honeydew melon

½ lemon, plus 1 tablespoon lemon juice

½ medium cucumber

1 teaspoon spirulina powder

Juice spinach, melon, lemon, and cucumber into a glass. Add the spirulina powder and lemon juice, then whisk well to combine.

Juice up this super immunity-boosting lemonade when you're not feeling so hot. Whisk in some spirulina or green superfood if you're in need of an extra jolt of immunity!

SERVES 1 ▶ **PER SERVING** 100 CALORIES | 1 G FAT | 6 G PROTEIN | 22 G CARBOHYDRATES | 0 G FIBER | 17 G SUGAR | 90% DV VITAMIN A | 130% DV VITAMIN C | 25% DV IRON | 10% DV FOLATE

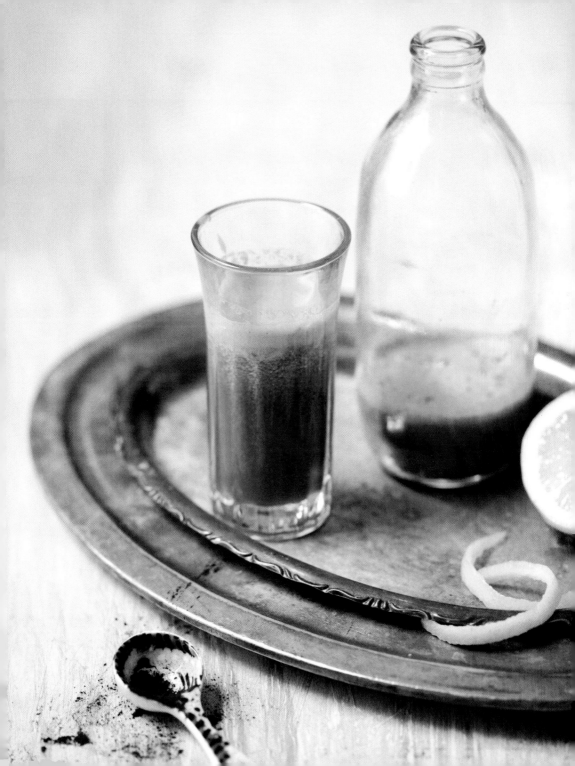

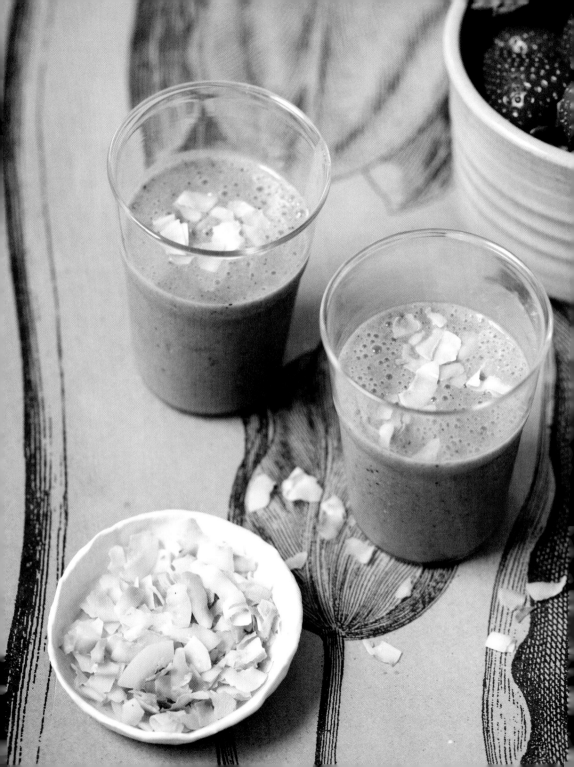

THE STRAWBERRY TOASTED-COCONUT IMMUNITY

SMOOTHIE › STRAWBERRY, COCONUT, LEMON

2 **cups unsweetened coconut milk drink**

2 **cups organic frozen strawberries**

2 **tablespoons toasted coconut shavings (divided)**

1 **tablespoon lemon juice**

1 **tablespoon spirulina (optional)**

1 **teaspoon bee pollen**

Combine ingredients and one tablespoon of the coconut; blend until smooth. Toast remaining coconut shavings in the upper third of the oven for a few minutes at 350°F. Let cool, then top smoothie with toasted coconut.

Sometimes you've gotta go pink! I developed this recipe for a bunch of my girlfriends who were stopping over for brunch; and I had to add a sexy topping to these smoothies. Why not toasted coconut? Tart strawberries, coconut milk, and delicious toasted coconut–this recipe was born to please.

SERVES 4 ▶ **PER SERVING** 70 CALORIES | 4 G FAT | 1 G PROTEIN | 10 G CARBOHYDRATES | 3 G FIBER | 4 G SUGAR | 60% DV VITAMIN C | 15% DV VITAMIN D | 6% DV FOLATE

THE SUPER CHARGER

JUICE › ROMAINE, CARROT, GINGER, LEMON

1 **head romaine lettuce**

3 **organic carrots, scrubbed**

1 **tablespoon fresh ginger**

¼ **tablespoon lemon juice**

Juice lettuce, carrots, and ginger into a glass. Then whisk in lemon juice to combine.

When in need of a cleansing kick in the A.M., I juice up this amazing glass of supercharged greens, carrots, ginger, and lemon and start feelin' good! The lemon can add a bitter taste, but learn to embrace the bitterness—it's naturally good for you.

SERVES 1 ▶ **PER SERVING** 110 CALORIES | 2.5 G FAT | 10 G PROTEIN | 21 G CARBOHYDRATES | 0 G FIBER | 15 G SUGAR | 710 MG OMEGA 3 | 2,160 MG POTASSIUM | 1,700% DV VITAMIN A | 70% DV VITAMIN C | 220% DV FOLATE

THE BLUEBERRY SUPER-IMMUNITY BOOSTER

SMOOTHIE › BABY SPINACH, GREEN SUPERFOOD, BLUEBERRY, BEE POLLEN

1½ **cups coconut water**

3 **cups baby spinach**

1 **tablespoon green superfood**

1 **frozen banana**

1 **cup frozen blueberries**

1 **teaspoon bee pollen**

1 **tablespoon spirulina**

Add ingredients into a blender and blend until smooth.

With a super-boost of spinach and anti-inflammatory blueberries, this smoothie has your health covered. Add in some extra green superfood or protein powder if you'd like.

SERVES 3 ▶ **PER SERVING** 120 CALORIES | 1 G FAT | 4 G PROTEIN | 27 G CARBOHYDRATES | 5 G FIBER | 13 G SUGAR | 510 MG POTASSIUM | 35% DV VITAMIN A | 20% DV VITAMIN C | 30% DV IRON

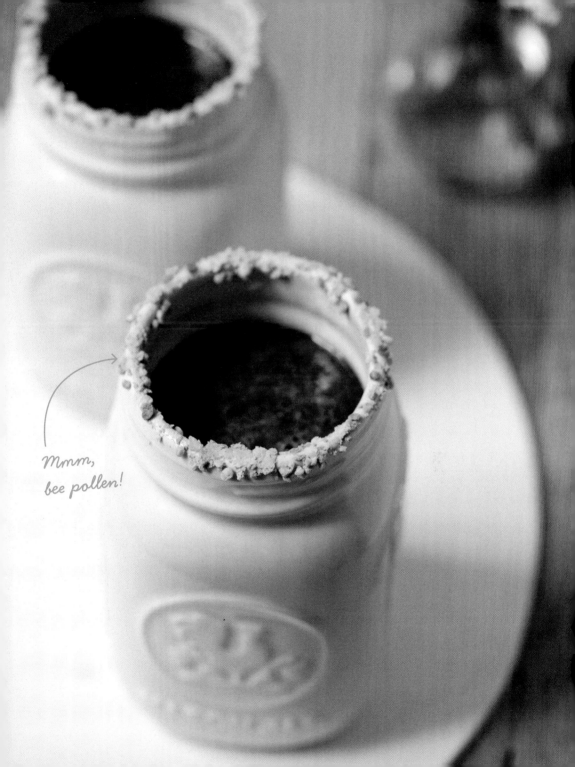

Mmm,
bee pollen!

THE VITAMIN C IMMUNITY BOOSTER

SMOOTHIE › STRAWBERRY, ORANGE, YOGURT

½ cup coconut water

1 cup frozen strawberries

2 oranges, peeled

1 cup Greek or coconut yogurt

1 tablespoon bee pollen

1 teaspoon probiotics

1 cup ice

Add ingredients into a blender and blend until smooth.

With refreshing strawberries and special immunity-boosting ingredients like bee pollen and probiotics, get ready for a magical blended surprise. And while you're at it, toss in some spinach and kale. Clean and Green.

SERVES 2 ▶ **PER SERVING** 120 CALORIES | 0 G FAT |
9 G PROTEIN | 22 G CARBOHYDRATES | 4 G FIBER | 15 G SUGAR |
120% DV VITAMIN C | 10% DV CALCIUM | 8% DV FOLATE

THE STRAWBERRIES &
CREAM IMMUNITY

SMOOTHIE ▶ BABY SPINACH, BANANA, STRAWBERRY

2½ cups unsweetened
   coconut almond milk

1 cup baby spinach

1 frozen banana

2 cups frozen strawberries

1 teaspoon probiotics

1 teaspoon bee pollen

Add ingredients into a blender
and blend until smooth.

Let's get that high fever down and your immunity up
with this delicious strawberry-blended smoothie.
Enjoy, gorgeous.

SERVES 3 ▶ **PER SERVING** 110 CALORIES | 2.5 G FAT |
2 G PROTEIN | 21 G CARBOHYDRATES | 4 G FIBER | 10 G SUGAR |
80% DV VITAMIN C | 40% DV CALCIUM | 20% DV VITAMIN D |
45% DV VITAMIN E

THE RECOVERY

SMOOTHIE ▶ KALE, BANANA, STRAWBERRY, BLUEBERRY, FENNEL SEEDS

1 cup unsweetened
   almond milk

1 cup kale

2 frozen bananas

1 cup frozen strawberries

1 cup frozen blueberries

1 tablespoon fennel seeds

1 cup ice

Add ingredients into a blender
and blend until smooth.

We all have those long Sunday mornings when we
wish we had skipped out on last night's final round of
Champers or red wine. But, hey, it was totally worth it,
right? And I wouldn't be able to create a killer recipe
like this if not for the occasional overindulgence.
Whip this up in the morning. Feel like a champ—truly.

SERVES 2 ▶ **PER SERVING** 110 CALORIES | 1.5 G FAT |
2 G PROTEIN | 24 G CARBOHYDRATES | 4 G FIBER | 12 G SUGAR |
35% DV VITAMIN A | 70% DV VITAMIN C | 15% DV VITAMIN E

THE GREEN ORANGE-GINGER

JUICE › CUCUMBER, BABY SPINACH, ORANGE, GINGER

½ large cucumber

3 cups baby spinach

1 orange, peeled

1 tablespoon ginger

Add all ingredients into a juicer and juice.

When you need a natural immunity boost, opt for this simple green OJ! With ginger's anti-inflammatories, orange's vitamin C, and spinach's phytonutrients, this super-juice will give you an organic boost of super-immunity! Who needs vitamin C packets and pills when you can go green?

SERVES 1 › **PER SERVING** 60 CALORIES | 0 G FAT | 3 G PROTEIN | 13 G CARBOHYDRATES | 0 G FIBER | 9 G SUGAR | 60% DV VITAMIN A | 100% DV VITAMIN C | 15% DV IRON

THE BERRY BEAUTY IMMUNITY

SMOOTHIE › BANANA, BLUEBERRY, STRAWBERRY, RESVERATROL

1½ cups coconut water

1 cup baby spinach

1 cup frozen blueberries

1 cup frozen strawberries

2 teaspoons spirulina

1 tablespoon probiotics/ acidophilus

2 tablespoons resveratrol

Add ingredients into a blender and blend until smooth.

If beauty starts from within, this is the perfect beverage for you to enjoy when you need to prop up your immunity and revive your beauty regimen. Fewer wrinkles and fewer colds; you're looking berry beautiful.

SERVES 3 › **PER SERVING** 80 CALORIES | 0.5 G FAT | 2 G PROTEIN | 18 G CARBOHYDRATES | 3 G FIBER | 10 G SUGAR | 360 MG POTASSIUM | 40% DV VITAMIN C | 6% DV IRON

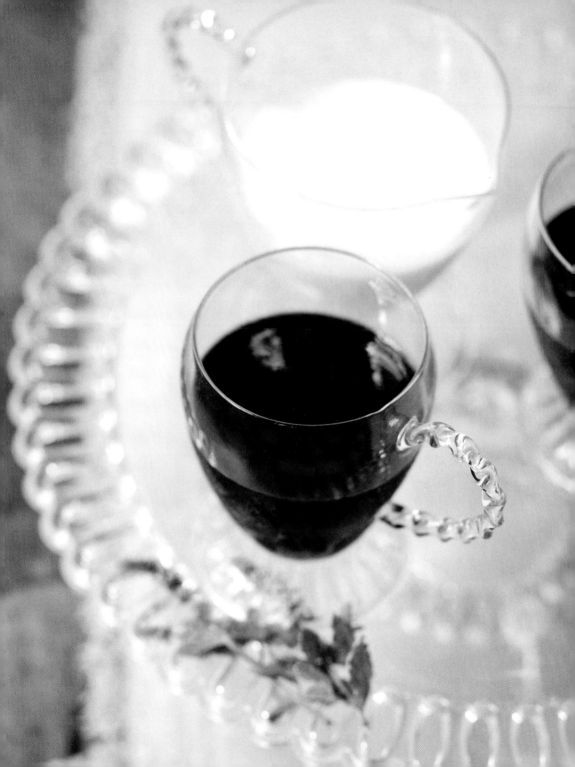

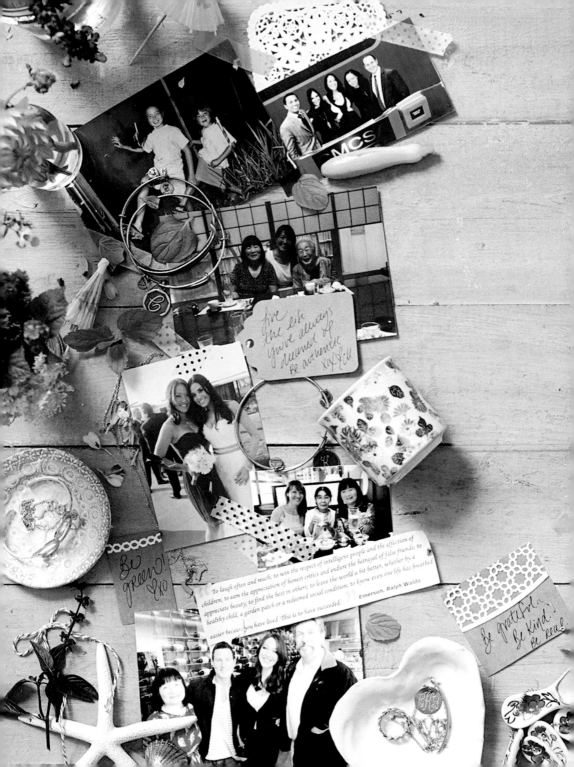

live
the life
you've always
dreamed of
be authentic
xx Jill

Be green! xo

Be grateful.
Be kind!
Be real!

To laugh often and much; to win the respect of intelligent people and the affection of children; to earn the appreciation of honest critics and endure the betrayal of false friends; to appreciate beauty; to find the best in others; to leave the world a bit better, whether by a healthy child, a garden patch or a redeemed social condition; to know even one life has breathed easier because you have lived. This is to have succeeded.   Emerson, Ralph Waldo

ACKNOWLEDGMENTS

As the years have gone by, I have realized that I am constantly immersed in light and love. I am so grateful to be surrounded by so many incredibly talented individuals. This was a collaboration of efforts between some of my nearest and dearest. A graceful, warm thank you…

To Mom, Dad, and Jenni, my life is so unique because you raised me to be independent through art, creativity, culture, and heart. Thank you for allowing me to dream so BIG. Dad, you have become one of my best friends this year. Thank you for opening up to me.

To Galvanized: Dave Zinczenko and Stephen Perrine. Some opportunities (and individuals) come only once in a lifetime. You have brought some of the greatest works to fruition thus far in my lifetime. Thank. You. I am beyond grateful and adore you both.

To AMI and David Pecker, thank you for the opportunities, kindness, and support you have created within your family. To Daniel Rotstein, Dina Zajicek, David Jackson, Liz Rutolo, Caroline Abba, Lawrence Bornstein, and Chris Polimeni, thank you!

To Cat Perry, Mike Smith, and Cecelia Smith, thank you for your kindness and your incredibly talented hard work and long days of edits and layouts. I am so grateful. Dearest Evi Abeler, you are such an incredible woman, mentor, and photographer. Thank you for your gorgeous work. Laurie Knoop, one of my favorite food stylists, thank you. Every day I am grateful I get to work with talented women like you! To Jade Rosenberg, you're such a light in my life. Thank you for every day! To Carla and Liz, my favorite art/prop/production ladies. Thank you for helping me to better "green" my life. I am so grateful for your talents.

Joe Heroun, your humility, talents, and grace make me want to work even harder. Thank you for being such a mentor. To Allison Zinczenko and John Hammond, from the moment I met you two I knew our relationships would grow into something beautiful. Thank you! To my lovely Danielle Praport, thank you for holding my hand for years. We grow together. To George Karabotsos, thank you for your hard work and Clean Green dedication. Brian Good, for all of your management. I'll be sure to rock my leather vest for you. ;) James Dimmock, thank you for such a gorgeous cover shot! To Samantha Irwin, thank you for your kindness. To Laura and Maureen, thank you for all of the edits, fact-checks, and notes. Wendy Hess, you are an incredibly hard-working R.D. Without you we'd lead without truth.

To the Clean Green shoot team: Seevon, Gloria, and Robert, thank you for always making me FEEL beautiful. I love you like my own family. Helenski, you are too talented with style! Christina, Deanna, Dina, Brooke, Sky, Rich, Priya, and Sharon Ryan! Thank you for all of your hard, beautiful work on the shoot! Love and hugs!

To my beautiful *Shape* ladies: Tara Kraft, Amanda Junker (you are amazing!), Locke, Abby, Britt, Alanna, and Heidi. Thank you for being so kind to me and helping me share my love for nutritious, beautiful food. I adore all of you gorgeous, hard-working editors. To my darling *Men's Fitness* team: John Rasmus, Dean Stattmann, Hollis Tempelton, Chris Hunt, and more, thank you for being so chill and FUN to work with.

To my Baachan, my Auntie Takuko, and the Kumai and Gwiazdowski families. I'm so proud of my Japanese-Polish heritage. We are resilient.

To Random House and Zinczenko/AMI Ventures, thank you! I am so grateful for all!

To my beloved agents at WME, thank you for holding my hand and heart: Justin Ongert, Strand, Googel, Bethany, Sherman, Amir, Kirby, Rosen, Wachs, Bider, Warner, EJ, Rob K., and all of the assists, especially Matt B. I love all of you. Xxo

To my best friends, this has been the toughest year; yet, I wouldn't have made it without you. Stephanie, I love you and miss you always. My CA girls: Christina, Casey, Andy, Suz, Tina, Michelle, Courts, and Dana. NY crew: Julie, Jenelle, Molly, Kat, Rico, and Barry, I love all of you and hold a very special place in my heart for you! To my Bar Method sisters: SD to SF, LA to my home in NYC/SoHo, thank you for being a family to me, my place of sanity. To all of my charitable partners, thank you for the opportunities. The James Beard Foundation, Chef's Garden, 1,000 Days, Health Corps, and UN Foundation. To my encouraging colleagues Kris Moon, Farmer Lee Jones, Simon Majumdar, Heidi Kristoffer, and Ellie Krieger.

To anyone who has ever made my recipes or read my books. May you be inspired to live a beautiful, fulfilling, whole life. Like, totally.

Finally, to the Big Man Upstairs: Thank you for every day. I am humbled by your grace.

Peace out, yo. Expect more greatness. xxCandice